"Joey does a great job of creating a straightforward, simple eating and lifestyle plan that doesn't chain you down to zero carbs, crazy supplements, or gimmicky exercises. `Fatness to Fitness' is an easy read and super simple to follow."

Christopher Guerriero
Bestselling Author, ``Maximize Your Metabolism"
www.MaxYourMetabolism.com

"Joey hit a home run with 'Fatness to Fitness.' I loved reading his story. It's intriguing and his practical advice is right on the mark. You will be inspired and informed at the same time. That is a winning combination for a best seller."

Victoria Johnson
Top Celebrity Trainer, Fitness Video Star
www.FemaleBodyMakeover.com

"Far from being just another diet book, 'Fatness To Fitness' is both a compelling and motivating autobiographical account of one man's real-life fitness journey, as well as a solid common-sense guidebook to living a healthy lifestyle and inspiring others to do the same."

Tom Venuto, NSCA-CPT, CSCS
Author of "Burn the Fat, Feed the Muscle"
www.BurnYourBodyFat.com

"Don't let the title fool you. This is not just a fitness book. Joey's advice will help you make the right choices for enhanced health, energy and happiness."

Jon Gordon
Author of the international best seller ``*The Energy Bus: 10 Rules to Fuel your Life, Work and Team with Positive Energy.*"
www.JonGordon.com

"In *'Fatness to Fitness*,' Joey Atlas skillfully blends his professional expertise with relatable personal accounts to deliver a sensible and informed approach to better health, nutrition and fitness. Well-written and to-the-point, this book is for anyone who wants lasting success with healthy eating and exercise."

Amanda Vogel
Certified Fitness Professional and Writer for *Health, Cooking Light, All You, SELF* and *Prevention* magazines.
www.ActiveVoice.ca

D1367303

"Great book! It is a great tool for clients like ours because it answers a lot of questions that I get asked all of the time. Far from a 'fad' way of thinking (which always makes us dietitians happy), the menus show the reader that it is possible to eat healthy without spending a ton of time in the kitchen preparing and cooking meals. I will definitely refer my clients to this book."

Jillian McMullen, RD, LD/N
Nutrition Consultant
www.JillianRD.com

"The mind-body connection is not to be underestimated and Joey beautifully demonstrates this to us in his book by emphasizing the importance of feeling good inside and out. The plan is simplified in a way that you can tailor it to your needs and desired outcome. And, like Joey, my favorite is the dark chocolate!"

Lisa Britt
Psychotherapist and Author of *"The Grateful Garden: How to Cultivate Gratitude and Bring More Joy Into Your Life"*
www.LisaBritt.com

"Joey's 'Fatness to Fitness' sends a message that is so often overlooked in training programs available today...that fitness is NOT limited to washboard abs and big bulging muscles. Our bodies are a direct reflection of how we feel about ourselves, respect ourselves, and even how seriously we take our commitment to our loved ones to be a good role model and to live long enough and healthy enough to enjoy them for years to come.

'Fatness to Fitness' takes you by the hand and guides you through all of the confusing information littering the weight-loss industry today, while blasting away all of the myths and obstacles that may have held you back in the past.

Joey's care, concern and commitment to your success drip from every page and it's like feeling he's there with you through your entire journey on the path to getting in the best shape of your life. Get this book! You'll live longer, healthier...and LEANER!"

Jeff Anderson
www.TheMuscularNerd.com

"Joey's new book is a must read for anyone wanting to get fit and STAY FIT ONCE AND FOR ALL! This practical information will be your guide as you make your journey towards optimal fitness a reality."

Tim Wambach
Author of *"Keep On Keeping On"*

"I've been in the fitness industry for 16 years now and have helped thousands of people from more than 100 countries around the world. I know what's good and what is not and I can honestly say that I recommend `Fatness to Fitness' without the slightest hesitation. Get a copy and take action now - you will not regret it!

"Fatness to Fitness" is so much more than just a book. It's a step-by-step guide to looking and feeling your very best. It's chock-full of sound advice, but in an easy-to-follow format that you can actually adapt to your busy schedule. I loved the lessons and I loved that it focused not only on nutrition and exercise, but also on how to have the right mind-set.

I think you'll find it very refreshing that Joey has been where you might be right now. He knows how you feel and he knows how to lead you to your best. He's been there and is ready to show you the way. With this book, you have a blueprint for success. All that's left is for you to take action. Take advantage of all that it offers and looks forwad to achieving your optimal self."

Chad Tackett, BS, CPT
President, Founder – Global Health and Fitness
www.YourFitnessPlans.com

"…very well-written with solid, common-sense (which isn't so common) information for the masses. The menus seem quite diverse, which for most people is a good thing.

If people follow it, they should see excellent results. I will be giving many of these recommendations a shot myself. In short, it's hard to fault a book that presents a diet full of mostly unrefined foods and healthy fats. The variance with the occasional bagel and other starchy foods makes the diet that much more acceptable.

The book is a bit short, but that may be a good thing. Great job, Joey! I enjoyed the read."

Jon Benson
Transformational Life Coach, Health & Fitness Counselor and
Award-winning Web Author – "*Fit Over 40*"
www.GettingFitOver40.com

FATNESS
to
FITNESS

*Former 'Fat Kid' Reveals His Most Powerful Personal
Strategies and Techniques to Help You Quickly and
Safely Achieve Permanent Fitness Success*

By Joey Atlas

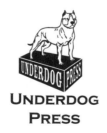

**UNDERDOG
PRESS**

Fatness to Fitness

For information, write to Underdog Press, 1637 Race Track Road, St Johns, FL, 32259; or call (904) 436-6052.

DISCLAIMER
This book includes information from many sources and from many personal experiences. It is published for general reference and is not intended to be a substitute for independent verification by readers when necessary and appropriate. The book is sold with the understanding that neither the author nor the publisher is engaged in rendering any medical, health, psychological or legal advice. The publisher and author disclaim any personal liability, directly or indirectly, for advice or information presented within. Although the author and publisher have prepared this manuscript with the utmost care and diligence and have made every effort to ensure the accuracy and completeness of the information contained within, we assume no responsibility for errors, inaccuracies, omissions or inconsistencies. The reader should consult a physician before acting on any advice contained in this book.

ISBN 978-1-60530-515-8

Quantity discounts are available to companies, educational institutions and fitness/wellness organizations for resale, educational purposes, subscription incentives, premiums, gifts or fundraising campaigns.

For information, please call:
(866) 937-5639

To my wife, Jeri-Jo, and my children,
JoJo, Alexa and Darah for their constant support and
for dealing with me "always being on that computer."

I love you guys…

Acknowledgments

Special thanks to:

My family and friends for helping me develop
"the tools" to always push forward and never quit.
Thanks, mom and dad, for EVERYTHING.

My editor, Tracy Carbasho – who went way beyond
the duties of editor to help me get this book done. If
you need a great editor, contact her at tcarbasho@earthlink.net
or (304) 312-9523.

Fitness colleague, Amanda Vogel, whose ``down-the-stretch''
input and advice took this book up at least several notches.

Mike Letis, my first client, mentor and friend, whose valuable
life and business lessons would not have been learned anywhere
else. Mike, you've made a huge impact on my life.

All of my clients around the world – past, present and future.
I sincerely thank you for your support and loyalty. Be Fit!

Fatness to Fitness
Table of Contents

Introduction

The journey to overall fitness of mind, body and spirit often has many twists and turns, but do not be discouraged. Sometimes, reaching our goal simply requires us to embrace the road less traveled by being true to ourselves and remaining focused on the ultimate goal of improving our overall wellbeing. Staying the course can be difficult in a world where we are continually inundated with compelling advertisements for yet another trendy diet, one more weight-loss pill or a new workout craze. The majority of these advertisements promise results, but do not provide the necessary tools to achieve the specified outcomes.

This book is designed to give you practical advice that will make it easy for you to reach your fitness objectives. You do not need expensive equipment, you do not have to travel to a specialty food store to buy hard-to-find ingredients for healthy meals and you do not have to spend hours in the gym every day.

I write these words with heartfelt sincerity as a former "fat kid" who has transformed his own life and has spent many years helping others realize their dream of lifelong fitness by using a common-sense approach. The lessons I learned about how to develop an effective exercise and nutrition program are rooted in my childhood and the influence of my father, whose Sicilian parenting methods were a bit unconventional.

I vividly recall one particular bonding experience between me and my father that was more suited for an episode of a quirky sitcom than the pages of Parenting magazine. I was sitting at the dinner table with my parents, my grandparents, my brother and my sister. They were enjoying a traditional Italian meal of pasta and peas, but I was determined to walk away from the table without taking one bite. My father had told me repeatedly to eat my dinner and I persistently replied that I did not like peas and, therefore, I was not eating the meal.

My father, who was just as obstinate, finally gave me an ultimatum. If I didn't start eating by the time he counted to five, he was going to dump the entire plate of food on my head. "One, two, three... " When he reached the final number, I still had not lifted my fork and my father proved he is a man who keeps his word. He poured the food on my head, sat the bowl on top of my head like a hat and then gave it a few side-to-side turns to rub it in.

To my father's surprise, I stated, "Good because now I don't have to eat it." In retrospect, perhaps I made a poor judgment call by being so bold at the age of ten. My father then led me to the stove and tried to feed me directly from the large pot with a metal serving spoon, still trying to explain that it was important for me to eat my dinner. All the while, my family is finding humor in our exchange and my grandmother begins to yell in her Italian dialect for my father to stop wasting the food.

Even though I wasn't aware of it at the time, I learned a valuable lesson that day. It would be years later before I would reflect back upon that family meal, but I believe it formed the foundation of my philosophy about helping others enhance their health. Samuel Butler, a 19th Century novelist, expressed it eloquently when he wrote, "A man that complies against his will is of his own opinion still." In other words, you cannot force someone to follow your advice or subscribe to the same philosophy about exercising and eating well. People will only do what they truly and genuinely want to do.

I intend to help you discover your own potential by creating a mindset where fitness becomes a byproduct of how you live your life every day and not a goal you grudgingly force yourself to work toward. My hope is that exercising and eating healthy meals will become as innate to you as brushing your teeth. Regardless of whether you are a fitness beginner, a professional trainer or someone who falls in between, my program will assist you in defining realistic goals and outlining a plan of action to achieve those objectives.

And in case you are wondering, not only have I grown to enjoy peas, but I also crave them occasionally. At least twice a week, I'll open a can of organic peas, drain the water, add a tablespoon of olive oil with some black pepper and eat it for lunch.

Nutritional stats:

365 total calories
14 grams of natural protein
10.5 grams of healthy fiber
Only 42 grams of nutrient-dense, high-quality carbohydrates (10 from the fiber)

You do the math…

CHAPTER ONE:
How to Make Your Food Work For You, Not Against You

As a short, pudgy child, I never imagined I would one day grow up to compete in bodybuilding competitions and win the title of Mr. SUNY Buffalo at the age of 20. Even more shocking is the fact that two days after capturing the title, my entire body was bloated from embarking on a ravenous eating binge. This was the beginning of a sickening downward spiral that was so out of control I truly thought I was going to die.

A vicious cycle took hold of my life when I started to participate in bodybuilding competitions while attending the State University of New York (SUNY) at Buffalo. For two months prior to each competition, I would keep a tight handle on my caloric intake, stay away from junk food, do intensive weight training and include approximately an hour of cardiovascular exercise in my daily workouts. The strict diet and rigorous exercise program were effective at bringing my body fat down to 2.8 percent and my weight down to 127 pounds.

However, this marked the first time in my life that I had actually deprived myself of my favorite foods, such as bread, muffins, cakes, chocolate and ice cream. It was brutal, especially for a former fat kid who was born into an Italian household where food was considered part of the cultural heritage. All of our family gatherings centered around eating multiple-course meals and if you failed to eat a second helping, everybody noticed. "Mangia, mangia," which in Italian means "eat, eat," would have been an appropriate slogan for my family. And mangia I did.

This calorie-driven tradition, combined with my love for carbohydrates and anything containing chocolate, earned me a few unwelcome titles. I remember being called "fat kid," "porky," and of course, "pudgy." I was so self-conscious about being overweight as a child that I was the loner who would never go in the pool at summer camp.

Finally, I began to notice positive changes in my body during the sixth and seventh grades when I became more active and started participating in soccer, baseball and other school sports. I started to lose the flab and in its place, I began to see some muscle definition. I was so encouraged that I continued to be physically active in high school as I added martial arts and weight training to my exercise regimen. Since I was burning a high number of calories by doing painstaking workouts, I continued to consume a correspondingly large amount of food. My body composition was fine and I felt extremely good about myself. This seemingly positive streak continued right into college until competitive bodybuilding became part of my world.

While I was dieting to ensure top physical form for the competitions, I was simultaneously stockpiling all of my favorite foods and asking my mom to have some of her delicious home-cooked meals ready the day after each competition ended. In fact, the meals that I wanted to eat after each competition were planned two weeks in advance. My love for food never diminished, not even while I was depriving myself in the weeks before competitions. When a competition ended, the binging would start and I would gain as much as 11 pounds in two days. At one time, I weighed a whopping 150 pounds, a dangerous number for someone who is just slightly more than 5 feet tall.

This vicious cycle of unhealthy binging would begin immediately after every competition and would not stop until I was literally too nauseous to take one more bite. Even though I successfully prepared for each competition, it was clear that food still ruled me. I did not realize it at the time, but in retrospect I can understand my actions. I was not just treating myself to the food I was craving during my preparation for a bodybuilding event. Rather, the former fat kid was still fulfilling his desire and, even more so, his psychological need for food.

There was definitely some irony and a bit of hypocrisy in my life at that time. After all, I was working hard to earn a degree in exercise physiology with the ultimate career goal of being able to counsel and coach people about improving their health through proper exercise and nutrition. I had all of the answers, but I was still eating to the point of sickness. I was obsessed with food and I was living a life that was the antithesis of a true fitness lifestyle.

I received my bachelor's degree in exercise science from SUNY in 1992, started my personal fitness training business, got married and became a father. Before getting married, I weighed approximately 145 pounds and had never fully faced my "former fat kid" issues. A challenging work schedule, a bad automobile accident in 1995 and a stressful marriage that eventually ended in divorce brought my internal fat kid out of the shadows and back to the forefront. I became dependent upon food as a coping mechanism during stressful times and my weight climbed to 168 body-crippling pounds.

I had the necessary knowledge about physiology to realize what was happening to my body and I could feel all of the aches and pains that accompanied being overweight. Still, I felt powerless to stop the cycle.

Fortunately, I reached a point where I was reduced to wearing gray, drawstring sweatpants because nothing else fit. That was a valuable awakening for me and until then, food topped the list of priorities in my life. This was not the lifestyle I wanted and it was time for me to define my values. Did I want to be fat or did I want to be fit? I chose to be fit and I knew my life was going to change once I said goodbye to the former fat kid.

I defined my goals and decided that I wanted to be in control of my thoughts, emotions and actions; assume full responsibility for my health; and be a "practice what I preach" type of fitness professional for my clients.

My ordeal was a major revelation in helping me understand how people's mindset, their emotional fortitude and their life experiences can impact their ability to maintain a healthy lifestyle. Overeating during stressful times or as a reaction to an event is a very common coping mechanism. Using food to replace something that is missing in our life is an easy way to exercise control over the amount of pleasure we experience. When other area's of life are uncontrollable, food and the act of eating make us believe there is still something that we can manage.

A co-dependency develops when food becomes a person's primary source of pleasure and happiness. Most people are not even aware they are relying upon this destructive coping method. It just seems natural to eat whenever we feel a void, whether it is a real or imagined empty space in our daily lives. As this unhealthy habit continues, food becomes an emotional crutch that slowly erodes the health and optimal performance of the body, mind and spirit.

Understanding how food can be a friend or foe is essential to overcoming this crippling dependency. Only then, can you fully grasp the importance of maintaining a healthy diet.

CHAPTER TWO:
The Most Important Chapter in the History of Fitness Books

You have the universal right and the ability to be as fit as you desire within reason. Read that statement one more time and think about what it means. Many people in this world are unfit and unhealthy because they are not familiar with this universal law. Yet, most people probably would not believe this simple statement because it just sounds too good to be true. I assure you, though, that my personal fitness journey and the stories of countless people throughout the world who have been trained, counseled or coached by me demonstrate the power of this universal law.

Before embarking on your own journey, however, you need to ask yourself a straightforward, but powerful, question. What are my values? This one overriding question has many facets and must be answered honestly in order to put yourself in the appropriate state of mind to move forward. If you value the gift of life that you have been granted, it will be easier for you to make every day as healthy and enjoyable as possible.

People want to look good, feel fit, be toned and be sexy. While this superficial physical motivation is not wrong, it is a grossly imbalanced way of aiming for the goal of optimal fitness. It should be about more than solely what you see in the mirror. For example, I believe it is extremely important to be around for your loved ones for a long time and to not be a burden on them by letting your strength and vitality diminish with age. Do you want to set a priceless example for those around you, especially your children, about what it means to be thankful for life and to get the most out of it?

Personally, I want to set an invaluable example for my family members, my friends and other individuals who look to me for advice. Being a role model may sound like a daunting task, but the effort is easier than you think and it pays off with big rewards. Improving your own health may influence your spouse, children, parents, friends or colleagues to strive toward a similar goal and before you know it, a sequence of positive events has been set into motion.

I have seen this ripple effect firsthand and I thank my father for exposing me to the world of fitness at a young age. I remember my first visit to the gym like it was yesterday, although it was more than 30 years ago when I was only 5 years old. My father had just joined a new gym that was closer to our home, making it easy for him to work out on the weekends. The owner was kind enough to let me join my father when the gym was not crowded.

From the moment I stepped into the weight training room, I was completely mesmerized. Watching the men push and pull heavy weights with flawless form was an incredible sight to witness. Their physiques were similar to those of the superheroes I enjoyed watching on television every Saturday morning. The only difference was that these were real people.

The seed was planted and I told myself that when I grew up, I wanted to lift big weights and look just like my father and the other men in the gym. Of course, I have grown to understand that the pursuit of better health and fitness has a much deeper meaning than just lifting heavy weights and having bulging muscles. When I refer to fitness success, I do not mean just losing weight and looking better. Much more than that, I want you to experience the compelling impact you can have not only on all aspects of your own life, but also on the lives of the individuals around you.

My father taught me the importance of this universal law and now my children are learning from the healthy habits exercised on a daily basis by me and my wife, Jeri-Jo. My son, JoJo, and my daughter, Alexa, who are 11 and 9 years old, respectively, already enjoy exercising and usually snack on nuts and fruits instead of candy and cookies. Even my 3-year-old daughter, Darah, shows an interest in fitness by playing on the exercise ball and stretching.

I am sharing stories about my life to explain how the choices we make can positively influence other people. Choosing a healthy way of life will inspire others to follow suit by taking better care of themselves. However, before you can set an example, you must first assume responsibility for your own health and fitness. I will give you the necessary guidance to create a sensible action plan and help you understand why your previous exercise and diet programs may have failed.

As I mentioned in the introduction, the three fundamental elements of fitness are the mind, body and spirit. The mind, or mental aspect, of fitness is easy to understand, but the spirit part may require an explanation. Just like we have a mouth and nose, we also have a spirit. The only difference is that we cannot see our spirit because it is physically intangible, but we all have one. It's how we connect to the world around us. The thoughts you have, the words you speak and the actions you take are your spirit at work.

To put this into better perspective, consider that oxygen, carbon, hydrogen, nitrogen, calcium and phosphorus make up about 99 percent of the human body. The other one percent consists of a combination of about 20 elements, such as potassium, vanadium, zinc and sulfur. There is nothing special or extraordinary when you look at these elements individually. However, when all of these elements are combined in certain amounts and magically infused with the spark of life, known as the spirit, the human body is no longer just a mass, but rather a living, breathing, ultra-dynamic creation with unlimited potential.

Your spirit exists whether you are a spiritual person or not. Just for the record, let's not confuse spirituality with religion. No matter what your belief is about how we got here - whether by evolution, creation or a combination of both, it is your obligation to protect the gift of life you have received. The results of neglecting this obligation can be seen every day. Medical facilities are being stretched to the limit in terms of patient volume, health insurance costs continue to rise at staggering rates and the prescription drug industry is raking in massive profits because of the "personal neglect syndrome."

Think about your inner circle of family members, friends and colleagues. How many of them suffer from medical conditions? How many are on a program of regular exercise and wise nutritional habits? You also may ask these same questions in reference to your own health and habits.

Too many people live in poor health and are under the false impression that they are not supposed to be ill, even though their lifestyle habits are not conducive to being healthy and fit. I acknowledge that certain medical abnormalities and diseases are a fact of life and occasionally we will hear of the fitness or health fanatic who had a heart attack and died at a young age. However, a case like this is extreme and rarely happens in the general population. Of course, this type of occurrence makes for great media material, but the truth is that you are more likely to hear news media reports about the dire consequences of an unfit existence. We hear these reports on such a consistent basis that maybe society has become numb to the messages. Just a thought.

With so much publicity about what can happen if we do not exercise and eat properly, it is hard to imagine that numerous people still do not put fitness at the top of their priority list. Instead, they place their faith in doctors and take medicine with the hope of correcting the damage created by neglecting their mind, body and spirit. Neglect of the self results in weight gain, high cholesterol levels, elevated blood pressure, bone degeneration, diabetes, joint dysfunction, cardiovascular disease, muscle atrophy and a long list of other physical and psychological ailments.

Most people think of these health problems as normal effects of aging, genetics or just plain bad luck. In reality, they are warning signs of a poor lifestyle, bad habits and unhealthy choices. Certain conditions can be prevented, greatly reduced or controlled not just by what we eat or the type of workouts we do, but also by how we think. Your state of mind is the gatekeeper to permanent fitness success of the mind, body and spirit.

The fact that your mind, body and spirit work together can be used to your tremendous advantage. All three facets of your wellbeing are connected by your conscious and subconscious thoughts. Your spirit connects you to the unlimited powers of the universe and it is up to you to harness this energy and use it to achieve success. Doing so is not as esoteric as it may seem. Rather, it merely means exhibiting a proactive consciousness in your daily habits as you remember to exercise regularly and make healthy meal choices that are within your caloric needs.

The more you do this, the easier it will be to understand that fitness isn't just about looking good, but more importantly about defining your values and directing your thoughts and actions to be in line with those values. This intangible aspect of your fitness success relies on you empowering and strengthening your spirit by communicating with your "self."

Later in the book, I'll talk about "being your own personal trainer." One of the essential elements of achieving this is through the conversations you have with your self -- either quietly in your own mind or out loud as if you are speaking to a close friend. This is where big changes take place. This is how I went from " fatness to fitness."

CHAPTER THREE:
Deadly Myths and Ridiculous Misconceptions That Prevent Your Fitness Success

Developing the mindset necessary to enhance your overall health begins with rethinking what you currently believe about exercise and nutrition. Doing this simple mental exercise will help you change your belief system regarding the likelihood of reaching the level of fitness and health that is most suitable for you.

Unfortunately, numerous myths and misconceptions about exercise and nutrition have created widespread confusion and a subsequent lack of fitness success in the general population, a problem I refer to as The Fitness Failure Epidemic. On the next few pages, I will dispel these falsehoods to clear the way for a clean mental slate upon which we will place the foundation of your new belief system.

Myth Number One: *In order to be fit, I must have good genetics.*

Myth Buster: Good genetics is a widely misused term. In short, your genetics are what you make of them. It is not possible for all men to look like Mr. Universe or all women to look like Miss America because we all possess a vast range of genetic variations.

People who engage in self-destructive behavior naturally gravitate toward a long list of negative outcomes, such as obesity, illness and a poor emotional state. On the other hand, people who engage in behavior conducive to good health, improved fitness and soundness of mind will find themselves in the good zone of their genetic range where they will experience a favorable body composition, a better health profile and a happier, more energetic spirit.

In my opinion, bad genetics is merely an excuse for not being healthy rather than a proven scientific reason for certain people not achieving a realistic level of fitness.

Myth Number Two: *In order to become and stay fit, I have to spend 2 ½ hours at the gym every day.*

Myth Buster: This false notion has been around since the early days of fitness. Most people take their cue from other individuals who are not qualified fitness professionals. They mistakenly base their own perception about what they must do in order to get into shape on their observation of individuals who appear to be in peak health. The sad reality is that millions of people spend more time exercising than necessary as a direct result of being exposed to the inappropriate belief that fitness success requires an unrealistic time commitment. In turn, when others learn about this challenging time commitment of physical exertion, they inherently discount themselves from even having the ability to participate in a fitness program of their own.

Optimal fitness can actually be achieved by completing a 30- to 50-minute workout four to seven times per week, especially if you follow the sound nutritional habits outlined in this book. Fitness is essentially a byproduct of how you think and what you put inside your body and not a derivative of how hard and how long you exercise. Fitness is a state of being, not doing.

Myth Number Three: *I'm not a "fitness person" and exercise* *just isn't for me.*

Myth Buster: Taking care of yourself by exercising and maintaining healthy lifestyle habits should be an intrinsic aspiration, not a burden. Your body, mind and spirit require exercise in order to function with vigor, strength and flexibility. Each of us has been blessed with the gift of life, so we must utilize our full potential instead of letting our bodies wither away, our minds become idle and our spirits become disheartened.

Myth Number Four: *I am not overweight and, therefore, I do not need to exercise.*

Myth Buster: First-rate fitness and health are not dependent upon weight. Although weight is a critical element in everyone's fitness profile, it is only one factor and it cannot determine what a complete fitness profile may look like. There are numerous health parameters that cannot be seen without testing. For instance, bone density, cholesterol and blood pressure, to name a few, can still be at potentially deadly levels, even if you are not overweight. The good news is, however, that proper nutrition and exercise habits can often reverse certain health conditions that result from lack of exercise or a poor diet.

Men and women who are not overweight, but still out of shape, typically complain about being flabby, feeling weak, suffering from joint stiffness and not having enough energy. These are the telltale signs of a lifestyle without a fitness plan. Regardless of weight, we all need exercise and proper nutrition.

Myth Number Five: *Exercise is too dangerous for me. I know a lot of people who have been injured as a result of exercising.*

Myth Buster: Most people start a fitness program without proper guidance and instruction. Too often, the outcome of this blind undertaking does lead to injuries, which are sometimes serious. You cannot embark on your fitness quest by performing the same exercises you did years ago or by imitating what you see other people doing.

Ideally, you should seek the assistance of a qualified fitness professional, especially if you are just starting an exercise program. Guidance is available in many forms ranging from books and DVDs to one-on-one personal consultation and training by a professional. Videos and DVDs are perfect for exercise instruction because they make it much easier to follow proper form and progression. In addition, they create an atmosphere of having a professional instructor working out right beside you.

No matter what instructional method you choose, be sure to perform only exercises that are appropriate for your age and your level of fitness. For example, a 50-year-old former high school football player with a bad knee and an injured shoulder should not be engaging in high-intensity power-lifting routines. A person with this type of profile would be better suited following a program focused on core strengthening, full-body flexibility and simple body weight exercises.

Myth Number Six: *If my calories are too low, my metabolism will shut down and stop me from losing weight and possibly cause me to gain weight.*

Myth Buster: Ponder this. Have you ever seen photos or videos of overweight hunger strike participants? The human body is capable of functioning with the consumption of far less calories than most people devour on a regular basis. The equation is simple: If more calories are being burned for fuel than are being consumed, a caloric deficit occurs. Your body compensates for the deficit by honing in on the sources of fat storage. It is very rare that metabolic shutdown causes weight gain or the inability to lose body fat. This myth is more of a marketing tactic than a realistic weight-loss principle.

There are several other factors that are more likely culprits in causing the body to have difficulty in shedding excess pounds. These factors include water intake, sleep patterns and the miscalculation of one's true caloric intake, as well as over-the-counter and prescribed medications. Perhaps this metabolic mystery is more of an excuse to overeat while pursuing fitness.

Myth Number Seven: *I'm too old to be in shape.*

Myth Buster: Being old is the best reason to be in shape. What most people dismiss as being side effects of aging can be stopped and often reversed through proper nutrition and exercise. To put this into perspective, being in shape as a mature adult does not mean partaking in next summer's "hottest body" contest at the beach.

Rather, being in shape as a mature adult means maintaining the highest possible level of physical, spiritual and mental independence. Strength, balance, coordination and a reasonable body weight are just a few factors that can impact your level of independence as you age. Ask yourself this. Do you want your grandchildren pushing you around in a wheelchair or would you rather be chasing them around the park and doing all of the fun things they want you to do as a grandparent?

Regrettably, any or all of these myths can become reinforcements for the subconscious, allowing people to let themselves off the hook without guilt. I am living proof that anyone, even fitness professionals, can fall victim to mistaken beliefs. Fortunately, I am also a prime example of how we can work to overcome obstacles and rebel against misconceptions that are bad for our health.

When I was in my late teens and early 20s, I competed in a series of bodybuilding competitions. My life was consumed by the bodybuilding industry, which I can define as a cult from firsthand experience. I did what everybody else in this particular "crowd" was doing at the time. I worked out too much and literally planned my life around my exercise schedule and the bodybuilding competitions.

I accepted the aches and pains that accompanied the exhausting workouts as part of the territory, even though the discomfort was often unrelenting. Despite the agonizing pain, I would never entertain the thought of missing a workout for fear of losing one ounce of muscle mass.

I also spent a ridiculous amount of money buying muscle-builders, such as powders, pills and other proprietary formulas. In addition to working out too much, I ate too often and too much. The bodybuilding subculture has been trained to consume high-calorie diets to enhance muscle growth and prevent muscle breakdown. This gives the supplement industry a reason to market meal-replacement formulas, bars and shakes. The notion that you will build more muscle if you work out more and eat more sounds logical, but it is not.

As I got older, I began my fitness business and started a family. The challenge of devoting so much time to my workouts began to have a devastating effect on my emotions. Even though my lifestyle had changed and I had a family, I could not find a way to adjust my workout schedule. This cult was continuing to have a negative impact on all aspects of my life.

By now, you may be finding these details impossible to believe, especially about someone who now espouses the philosophy, "Don't be like everybody else. Be fit." I can understand your disbelief because I find it hard to imagine that the person I am describing was actually me. Thank goodness, that was a long time ago and I finally realized the biggest obstacles I had to overcome were in my head.

My problems were not being created by the demands of my business or my family responsibilities. I simply had to create a new approach that was compatible with my philosophy of a balanced and realistic approach to fitness. This did not happen overnight, though. It took me several years to develop a plan that enabled me to be fit and healthy, while enjoying my family and investing the necessary time in my fitness business.

The myths and misconceptions created by the bodybuilding subculture molded my mindset and prevented me from being able to comprehend the possibility of finding a better way of life. Reflecting on the transition I had to make in my own life helps me understand how people without a formal fitness education can get stuck in a bottomless rut and never find their way out.

Today, I receive emails on a regular basis from people around the world who are struggling to make the same transition, but they are often under the influence of a myth or misconception that has prevented them from moving forward. Now that I have dispelled these myths, it is time to take the next step by learning to overcome the obstacles that are preventing you from losing weight and being fit.

Before I end this CHAPTER, I do want to make note of the positive aspects of bodybuilding as they applied to my personal journey in life. First, it provided me with an "entry point" into the world of fitness and it got me hooked on taking action for self improvement.

In addition, it taught me the importance of mental/emotional power as it applies to personal change.

And lastly, it taught me the extreme importance of how "the things" we put into our bodies have a direct impact on the mind, body and spirit.

CHAPTER FOUR:
Mysterious and Frustrating Fitness and Weight Loss Obstacles

There are several factors that can interfere with your fitness progress or weight-loss goals. Quite often, these unobvious obstacles cause many people to throw in the towel and give up on their fitness quest out of sheer frustration and disappointment. Just knowing what these obstacles are is enough to tip the scales in your favor when things don't seem to be going right. Read on to learn about the most common offenders…

Fear and Guilt

Fear comes in many forms -- fear of failure, fear of rejection, fear of what your friends are going to think of the "new you," fear of how your spouse or companion is going to react, fear of having to stay committed to your new mindset and lifestyle. Guilt also has many faces -- guilt over being a little selfish (this is a healthy kind of selfishness), guilt over taking time for yourself and possibly away from your loved ones (not as bad as you being dead and gone forever), and guilt over changing how you (and maybe your family) eat.

That is just a small list of the many ways people can prevent themselves from achieving fitness success. These guilty feelings and fears can create a subconscious mindset that justifies not pursuing fitness and perpetuates the repeated experiences of fitness failure, often caused by self-sabotage.

This guilt and these fears can also provide the foundation for one's belief system and thought processes that reinforce a life lived without regard for one's optimal health and wellbeing.

Stacks and stacks of books have been written on fear and guilt, but I simply want to highlight them as potential reasons why you have not reached permanent fitness success. Sometimes, the mere recognition or admission of these psychological struggles can help a person take control of these feelings either by their own efforts or with outside professional guidance.

Stress and Sleep

There have also been numerous books written about sleep and stress. In order to stay focused on how they relate to your weight and fitness, I am going to keep this basic and straight to the point.

Stress has been part of life since the beginning of our existence and it always will be. That much I can guarantee. As perfectly crafted human beings, we have been given the amazing ability to handle random doses of stress at various levels with minimal impact on our wellbeing. It can also be argued that these typical life stressors make us even stronger as humans.

The evolution of society has created endless reasons for people to find themselves battling stress on a daily basis. This constant presence of stress can wreak havoc on the body. With its ability to affect various elements and hormones in the body, full-time stress can prevent the body from functioning at its best. The functions I refer to are the things we don't even have to worry about - functions that our bodies take care of by themselves. When certain elements get out of whack, however, the system starts malfunctioning and symptoms start to appear.

Irritability, low energy, weight gain, perhaps weight loss, and depression are some of the common symptoms of chronic high stress. Many studies have even shown death to be the direct result of chronic, intense stress. This is just another example of how one factor can cause weight gain, despite everything else being on the right track.

A similar relationship exists with sleep. During sleep, our bodies recuperate, repair and re-energize. This all happens incredibly by doing things at the most minuscule levels of our existence - a subject that ventures into the scientific realm, but is nonetheless crucial to our survival. Without adequate sleep, the body is prevented from experiencing all of the life-sustaining reactions that take place while we are in dreamland.

Poor sleep causes a chain reaction that touches so many parts of our routine functioning that symptoms can affect mental clarity, digestion, energy levels, basic metabolism, eyesight, sexual performance, muscle strength and mood to name just a few.

Prolonged high stress and lack of sleep can each be related to a weakening of the immune system and, hence, a threat to our overall health, not just our body weight or body composition.

The good news is that proper exercise and wise nutrition are easy ways to possibly cure or greatly alleviate your sleep and/or stress issues. Exercise helps you sleep better and is an outlet for stress, while a healthy diet provides the ideal elements needed "on the inside" for all of the reactions and processes that must take place throughout a 24-hour cycle.

Emotional Eating

The biggest problem here is that emotional eating is used to alleviate psychological hunger and not true physical hunger. In this context it becomes quite easy to understand how caloric intake can far exceed what is physically necessary to support life in the most optimal manner.

The key to ending destructive emotional eating is not to ask yourself, "How do I stop?" Rather, you should ask yourself, "How do I re-evaluate my life, my values and my desires to enable me to place priority on the things that are most important to me? How do I make sure my relationship with food is one that sustains and supports my life and not one that destroys it by serving as a coping mechanism to help me handle life?"

The true secret to conquering emotional eating is not by simply identifying situations and circumstances that trigger it, but by reframing your mindset so that you act in a favorable manner in those situations. You must remain in control of your thoughts and actions in a way that is completely in line with your true intentions.

Granted, there are some instances of emotional eating that require severe and strong intervention. For the general population, though, emotional eating can also be called "eating for happiness, stress relief and/or a sense of control in one's own life." In all cases, these feelings are short-lived and a co-dependency on food develops. This co-dependency is a very dangerous condition when combined with the amount of food and high-calorie beverages that are available to us whenever the desire arises.

I respect that no two situations are exactly the same and some cases may require more attention than I suggest. In my efforts to help the unfit and the "trying-to-be-fit" population, the main point I want to convey is that changing your mindset and defining your values can lead to a healthy co-dependency on health-promoting, energy-boosting, life-enhancing nutrition and exercise.

Prescription Medications

Weight loss and body-fat reduction present major challenges for most people who seek to achieve these goals. The challenge can often seem impossible to overcome when medication-induced weight gain is added to the mix. Prescription drugs are often overlooked as the culprit of unexplained weight gain or the inability to lose weight, despite being on a good program of wise nutrition and proper exercise.

There are many reasons why this problem goes unrecognized in the cases of countless people who suffer from this unwanted side effect. Quite often, the potential for weight gain as a side effect is not clearly noted in the printed materials and labels that accompany specific drugs. It is also likely that doctors may not be aware of weight gain as a side effect of a specific drug when writing a prescription for it. Likewise, if a drug is new to the market, it may not even be known that weight gain is a side effect in certain patients until actual usage reports start coming back to the pharmaceutical company that produces the drug.

There are also interaction side effects between certain drugs that may lead to weight gain, whereas, the drugs by themselves do not cause weight gain, but they may trigger this side effect when combined with other medications.

Now, we must understand that each person has a unique

biochemical profile, generally speaking. As a result, not everyone reacts the same to certain elements that are put into the body. However, there are certain groups of drugs that are known to cause weight gain in a certain percentage of patients who are taking one or more of them.

Certain prescription medications used to treat mood disorders, seizures, migraines, diabetes and high blood pressure can cause weight gain - sometimes up to 10 pounds per month. Some steroids, hormone-replacement therapy and oral contraceptives can also lead to unwanted pounds, even for people who are eating right and exercising on a regular basis.

Steroids, such as Prednisone; older antidepressants, such as Elavil and Tofranil; and second-generation anti-psychotics like Zyprexa are the most commonly recognized promoters of weight gain. Other common offenders include the antidepressants Paxil and Zoloft, the anti-seizure medication Depakote, diabetes drugs like Diabeta and Diabinese and the high blood pressure drugs Cardura and Inderal. Heartburn drugs like Nexium and Prevacid may also cause drug-induced weight gain.

An important note here is that it is not always the drug itself that is causing the weight gain. For example, antidepressants work to improve a person's mood and when the individual is feeling better emotionally, his or her appetite often increases. Therefore, the caloric intake is higher and if there is no increase in physical activity during this period, those extra calories show up in the form of body fat.

While some drugs used to treat depression and other mood disorders can cause weight gain, the antidepressants Wellbutrin and Prozac tend to help people lose weight. Some medications used to treat seizure disorders and headaches, such as Zonegran and Topamax, are known alternatives that are both associated with weight loss.

Another side effect may be fluid retention and swelling. In this case, a drug causes the patient to store a higher capacity of water in areas of the body where fluids did not accumulate before the drug was present in the body. Some people describe this as having "soft and puffy" skin or having a constant bloated feeling.

There are various medications that can be used to treat the same ailment, but each may result in a different side effect. Again, biochemistry and some trial and error will play a part here. As long as you are aware of your starting point and note any changes you experience, you will have the necessary feedback to bring to your doctor's attention. The goal will then be to modify your dosage or switch to another medication, while still successfully treating your condition.

When starting to take any prescribed medicine, make it a priority to understand all of the potential side effects that can be caused by the drug. After you have read about the side effects or if you experience any of them, you may want to discuss alternatives with your doctor. Open lines of communication are important and you are responsible for being proactive regarding your medical needs and treatment options.

Thyroid Conditions

Located just below your Adam's apple is the thyroid gland. It only weighs about one ounce, but it is responsible for many life-dependent functions throughout the entire body. One of these functions, metabolism, is controlled primarily by the thyroid gland. Two conditions can result from a faulty thyroid, hyperthyroidism and hypothyroidism. The first is categorized by an over-active thyroid gland. The second, hypothyroidism, is defined by an under-active thyroid gland.

According to the American Association of Clinical Endocrinologists, about 27 million Americans are affected by thyroid disease and eight out of every 10 are women. It is estimated that as many as 18 percent of women are diagnosed with postpartum hypothyroidism. Yes, pregnancy can shake things up a bit.

Some of the symptoms of an under-active thyroid are sluggishness, fatigue, weight gain, muscle cramping, hair loss and irregular menstrual cycles. Symptoms of an over-active thyroid include unexplained weight loss, irritability, insomnia, anxiety, heat intolerance and hand tremors.

Treating these thyroid conditions can often be as easy as taking a prescription drug to help the thyroid function properly. Synthroid and Cytomel are two of the commonly prescribed medications for an under-active thyroid gland. Drugs used to treat an over-active thyroid are Tapazole and Propyl-Thyracil. Severe cases may require radioactive iodine therapy or surgical removal.

If you have been exercising and eating properly, but are not getting the expected results, it would be a good idea to consult your doctor to determine whether your thyroid gland is affecting your metabolism.

Miscalculation of Daily Calories

For the purpose of simplicity, I am going to keep this brief. The miscalculation of one's caloric needs is so easy to do that it is one of the main reasons people fail to achieve optimal body composition. Depending on what source you are getting your information from and in what context it is being used, a 1,700-calorie diet can be considered high by some sources and low by others. Of course, this can be quite confusing to the average person.

Here is what I have learned through my own research and by hands-on experience. When we look at the most successful diets, they tend to have daily caloric ranges that fall into the 1,600-to-1,900-calorie zone for men and the 1,300-to-1,600-calorie zone for women.

Let's assume a typical middle-aged woman comes across a diet plan that includes exercise and promotes the daily intake of 2,800 calories. I would be willing to bet that most women who follow this plan would do so unsuccessfully with poor results. Keep in mind there may be a few women who would find success on this plan as compared to how they were living before starting this program. However, the majority would not do well on this program. The same comparison can be used for men.

Now let's take this one step further. After we understand how many calories we are supposed to consume in one day, it's time to make sure we actually take in that amount and not more. Yes, calorie counting may be a little tedious in the beginning, but it will eventually become second nature. The key here is to really pay attention to your daily needs and then make sure that your food choices and portion sizes keep you inside your daily calorie zone. Doing so simply requires a little conscious effort.

CHAPTER FIVE:
The Dirty Truth About the Dietary Supplement Industry --- Antioxidants, Vitamins, Minerals and Other Supplements

Sometimes when I'm shopping, I walk down the supplement aisle just to see if there are any new products promising outrageous results. The labels and ridiculous claims on some of these bottles make me laugh because I know the implied results are beyond far-fetched. From supposed muscle builders to fat melters - the offerings are endless -- and every big seller eventually gets replaced by the next miracle substance.

The problem is the vast majority of the general public does not know all of the facts and many people are inclined to believe there is some validity to what they read on the labels of these products. The supplement industry is a multibillion-dollar business, so it's clear that people are purchasing these products. The reason the top sellers keep getting replaced by new products is that eventually people realize the old ones did not live up to their promises and once again, people pin their hopes on the next hottest item.

Don't get me wrong. I'm not entirely against the nutritional supplement industry. There may be some cases where a certain health deficiency or medical condition may be alleviated or improved with the use of a supplement. A multidisciplinary medical practitioner would be the best person to consult for this type of guidance.

While I am a big believer and advocate of deriving your nutritional needs from a clean, healthy diet, I see no harm in taking a daily multi-vitamin and mineral supplement, using certain herbs for general purposes or even consuming a healthy nutrition bar or drink when it makes life more convenient. As always, I opt for organic choices in these instances.

There are some useful products and credible companies in the supplement industry, but there is so much misleading marketing that the ultimate burden falls upon you, the consumer. It is important to understand the eye-opening summary of the "gray area" in the dietary supplement industry. Here is what you need to know.

From weight-loss aids to sports-performance enhancers, supplements are not subject to testing and approval by the Food and Drug Administration before they are marketed to consumers. It amazes me that so many people are not aware of this important information, but it is true, nonetheless. A company does not even have to supply the FDA with evidence of safety unless the supplement contains a new dietary ingredient that was not on the market prior to Oct. 15, 1994.

How is this possible? As a result of the 1994 Dietary Supplement Health and Education Act (DSHEA), the FDA regulates the dietary supplement industry via a post-market program. This basically means the FDA must monitor all products, but only after they have been released to the market, to ensure the public's safety. This is done primarily through the voluntary reporting of adverse reactions. Translation: The FDA waits for consumers, health and medical professionals, and supplement marketers to report adverse effects that result from using a certain product. Sounds pretty limited, doesn't it?

A product can go to market, be purchased by consumers and be used as the consumer wishes. The FDA will only take action to ban a supplement or particular ingredient if it receives enough reports of adverse effects, serious medical complications or deaths that result directly from using a particular product.

Here is another problem with the industry. Supplements that are useless and ineffective CANNOT be banned by the FDA unless they pose a significant health risk. To further illustrate my point, I'll give you a fictitious example. A company can create a simple mix of vitamins and herbs that has absolutely no health benefit and give it a catchy name like "SlimEasyShortcut." As long as the ingredients on the label are in the bottle and the advertising does not violate any laws of the Federal Trade Commission, the company can continue selling the ineffective product. No harm, no foul. Crazy, right?

When the laxity of the FDA and FTC regulations are combined with the desperate hope and naive trust of the general public, along with clever packaging and marketing tactics, you end up with a multibillion-dollar industry that needs to be reformed. A great book on this topic is "Muscles, Speed, and Lies: What the Sport Supplement Industry Does Not Want Athletes or Consumers to Know" by David Lightsey.

A word on the FDA. The FDA does all it can to keep up with the high volume of dietary supplement companies, but the agency is vastly outnumbered. The administration does what it can with the resources it has available. I could list several pages of product seizures, big-dollar fines and other regulatory actions, but more should be done. While the FDA does some good, it also does some things that I just can't understand.

The herbal sweetener stevia, for example, has been used in Brazil and Japan for decades as a natural sweetener and food additive with a clean history of consumption. However, in the United States, it is not even on the GRAS (Generally Recognized as Safe) list. It can only be used if the product it is being used in has the words "herbal supplement" on it. It can't even be labeled as a natural sweetener. Silly, but true. As a side note, one of my favorite brands is KAL Pure Stevia - Organic Extract.

What's interesting is that two major companies recently filed for more than 20 U.S. patents regarding stevia for use in foods and beverages. The fact that they are filing for patents on this herb means they will be chemically altering it. That, in turn, also means that you will never see me consuming the chemically altered version and I would advise you not to either.

At this point, you know my belief in deriving all of our nutrients from natural food sources instead of pills and powders, but I want to add some reinforcement to my philosophy. Whatever power created us had the infinite wisdom to create the exact foods that we would need for optimal health and nourishment. There are "ingredients" in our foods that come from the earth and may never be identified or isolated by scientists in the lab. Therefore, they can never be duplicated in a supplement. It is the unique, universally created compositions of the foods that were put on this earth that give us everything we need. The big question is whether you are doing everything you possibly can to ensure your diet is varied and balanced enough to get all of the nutrients required for a fit, healthy and energetic life.

When I read about these mega-concentrated, super-antioxidant supplements, I just shake my head because the antioxidants we need are present in so many of the foods that are within easy reach. It is that simple. Our creator was a genius beyond our comprehension -- a genius who then created the most perfect foods with the precise ratios and concentrations of all necessary nutrients to fuel our existence with minimal or no processing at all. Makes all the sense in the world.

With a fairly decent diet coming from mostly organic sources, you can get nearly all of the nutrients your body can process and use. A dash of simple supplementation is fine (organic sources preferred), but there is no need for anyone to spend hundreds of dollars a month for what you can get from the foods that the earth produces.

Remember, most products are marketed by fear. The consumer fears what they could be risking or missing if they do not take a certain supplement. Don't let your fear motivate your supplement intake. Let your common sense and trust in the foods that were specifically created for you be your guide as to what you need to optimally sustain a strong, healthy and energetic life.

CHAPTER SIX:
The Truth Revealed: Organic Foods and Artificial Sweeteners, Preservatives, Flavors & Colors

The True Benefits of Organic Foods and Beverages

Several years ago, Aaron Gottlieb needed 18 hours of sleep a day. A visit to his doctor pinpointed the cause of the chronic fatigue: the Epstein-Barr virus. Following the diagnosis, friends introduced Aaron to organic foods and a vegetarian diet. One year later, he was 80 pounds thinner and feeling incredibly well. The experience led him to dedicate his life to helping others eat right, too, and in 1997, Aaron and his wife Erica opened Native Sun Natural Foods Market on San Jose Boulevard in Jacksonville, Fla. (www.NativeSunJax.com)

The paragraph you just read can be found on Native Sun's Web site. The success of the first location has allowed Aaron and Erica to open a second location in Jacksonville. These stores are two of our favorite places to visit, explore and shop because each is loaded with incredibly healthy and tasty foods that are not yet easy to find in the regular chain supermarkets.

Aaron's life-changing experience is a simple and straightforward testament to the power of "clean" nutrition. Some people are quick to point out the higher cost of organic foods and beverages. There is also an ongoing debate about whether organic foods are actually better for us than non-organic products. Interested parties on both sides of the debate have produced an enormous amount of information to support their personal opinions. The deluge of advertising materials, testimonials and research studies can completely overwhelm the average consumer. In fact, sifting through the information to find the right answers can be so daunting that many individuals relinquish their search and continue to consume the same foods they have always eaten.

In order to make it easy for you to distinguish between the benefits of organic versus non-organic, I will offer my viewpoint as it applies to my philosophy on permanent fitness success. As I have already mentioned, our existence is no freak-of-nature accident. Having spent an entire summer dissecting a human body and learning in very fine detail how each system works in harmony with the others to support the miracle of life, I have a unique perspective on the human body. To call it the ultimate machine would be a massive understatement and, therefore, I will refer to it as the ultimate creation.

This ultimate creation could only be fueled and sustained by perfectly created foods and water. In other words, the abundant foods that we naturally take for granted could be considered an extension of the human body because they provide all of the nutrients, vitamins, minerals and trace elements in perfect proportions and concentrations that you would need for your entire lifetime.

The food and water provided by nature not only give us the energy to move and think, but they also nourish the building blocks that create new cells as old ones die. In essence, the old saying "you are what you eat" has some truth to it. I believe we do become what we eat and this brings me back to the debate over whether organic foods actually provide any benefits over their non-organic counterparts.

Essentially, what we eat becomes us.

All science and studies aside, the only thing I need is intuition to help me decide for myself. If I have a choice between two apples - one which was farmed organically and the other farmed with the use of chemical pesticides, artificial fertilizers and/ or sterilized via ionizing radiation - I will choose the organic apple. This is a simplified example of what I am trying to illustrate, but the principle is the same.

The point I want to stress is that organically produced foods are how nature intended them to be farmed. The more chemicals they are exposed to and the more treatments they undergo, the further away from their natural composition they get and the less ideal they become for optimal health and fitness.

Yes, there is a slightly higher cost attached to organic goods, but these costs are coming down as the market expands and demand rises. There are some little known places where organic foods can be purchased at discount prices. One of my favorites is Big Lots (www.BigLots.com), a retailer that provides surplus foods and discounted household items. Quite often, the store will have a handful of organic products on the shelves.

One telltale sign of the growing organic trend is Wal-Mart's effort to offer more organic foods to its customers as a vital ingredient in its initiative to "go green." Wal-Mart's sustainability initiative will not happen overnight and, likewise, your family going organic does not have to occur by tomorrow. You might start with one or two items, such as milk or salads, and gradually add more organic foods to your diet.

Some of our staple organic foods that are always available at Wal-Mart are organic milk, eggs, green tea, frozen or canned vegetables, hot and cold cereals, ground flax seed and sugar.

There are more, but there are too many to list here. The point is - you can easily put together a "mostly organic" nutrition plan while sticking to a budget.

Keep in mind that a diet consisting of 20 percent organic foods is better than a diet that is only 3 percent organic. Don't feel pressured to go to 90 percent organic within three days. Gradual progression is fine when making a shift in your nutritional habits.

The ultimate benefit of consuming organic foods and beverages is that no matter how the big debate ends, you can have peace of mind knowing you are not taking a gamble when it comes to ingesting foods that have been processed with harmful chemicals.

Many supermarkets are realizing the public demand for organic foods and beverages and are subsequently carrying more of these products. Some of these stores are Shop Rite, Safeway and Target to name just a few. If you are unsure if your favorite supermarket carries organic foods, all you have to do is ask. They will be happy to point out all of the organic products they are stocking for people just like you.

Are You a Human Lab Rat? Artificial Sweeteners and Other "Things"

As a drug-free competitive bodybuilder, my primary focus was to lower my body fat as much as possible to prepare for competition. This was achieved primarily through calorie control. For a while, I relied on diet sodas and other diet beverages to help keep my calories in the lean zone until I realized something was wrong. I started paying attention to the number of headaches I was suffering and I began pondering why I was getting bloated, despite following what I thought was a healthy diet and exercising daily.

No stranger to reading food labels and understanding how to research specific ingredients, the first place I looked was the diet beverages. My initial research produced two very different perspectives regarding the sweeteners used in diet drinks. One side stresses the research studies illustrating the association between chemically created sweeteners and various medical conditions, while the other cites the total safety of the no-calorie, patented sweeteners as approved by the FDA for human consumption.

I read countless articles and quickly realized that I had to decide what was best for me. Eventually, I stopped drinking the diet beverages that are chockfull of artificial sweeteners and quickly noticed that my headaches had subsided and I was no longer bloated. Mind you, I was still preparing for competition. Relying again on my infinite powers of logic and common sense, I decided that artificial sweeteners were not for me and I cut them from my diet forever.

It was not difficult to give up the diet drinks because many of them had an unpleasant, lingering after-taste. However, I wanted an alternative and began searching for one. During my many visits to health food stores, I was introduced to an herbal extract called stevia. This incredibly sweet extract comes in powder or liquid form from the stevia plant. There are entire books that herald the benefits of stevia, but there also has been a lot of controversy surrounding it for years. A quick online search will give you plenty of educational material to allow you to decide for yourself.

I made up my mind about 17 years ago and I've been using

stevia ever since. I use it in my tea, my cereals and my espresso. It is readily available at most health food stores and via the Internet. My family has been using an organic stevia powder for the last few years and we love it.

There is a ton of literature available on all of the topics I have mentioned. You can spend hours on the Internet and walk away from your personal research with no clear picture on whether or not these things that are allowed to be added to our foods are good or bad. I offer my personal perspective in an effort to make your choices a little bit easier.

There have been so many advancements and breakthroughs in the medical establishment in recent years and some of them are quite amazing to say the least. Yet, there are still baffling medical conditions and terminal diseases that have not been traced to any particular source as a cause. How do we explain these? Do they just happen for no reason? I don't believe so. I believe everything has a cause.

Based on what I know about the body, what I have seen, read and heard, and what I have experienced both personally and indirectly through others close to me, I believe certain substances we consume can cause long-term harm to the body. These substances are the ingredients that I choose not to consume.

Have you ever eaten or drank something only to have a strange sensation or reaction occur on your tongue, lips, cheeks or throat shortly after you have consumed the product? I used to frequently experience this odd sensation. Dried fruits and a few other food and beverage items that I regularly consumed seemed to cause this type of reaction.

After reading about food additive sensitivity and reported reactions to certain ingredients, I began to make the conscious effort to choose foods that had less artificial preservatives, flavors and colors. For instance, I began eating unsulphured dried figs, I cut down dramatically on cold cuts (lunch meats) processed with nitrites and I stayed away from foods and beverages preserved with sodium benzoate. I started to become more mindful of artificial flavors and artificial colors, opting for foods and beverages without these ingredients.

Amazingly, the more adjustments I made, the less I experienced these weird sensations on my lips and in my mouth and throat. Very cool! And, of course, this experience got my mind to thinking about other related factors. If some of these agents can cause such abnormal reactions on the outside of my body, then what are they doing to the inside of my body? Could they be adversely affecting the internal systems of my body and causing problems that may take years to show up in the form of symptoms or a full-blown disease? There are two schools of thought here and both have evidence to back up their positions. Again, you must decide what makes sense and how you will proceed.

Here are some of the ingredients that me and my family avoid:

Artificial Sweeteners:

* Sucralose;
* Aspartame;
* Saccharin;
* Acesulfame Potassium;
* Cyclamate (banned by the FDA in 1969, but may be back on the market soon).

Artificial Preservatives:

* Sulphites (sulfur dioxide);
* Benzoates (sodium benzoate). Many companies are now removing this ingredient from their products.

Artificial Flavors:

* Monosodium glutamate (MSG). Known as a flavor enhancer;

NOTE: In 1995, the FDA acknowledged that some people may experience short-term reactions to products containing MSG. These reactions can include headaches, facial pressure or the sensation of skin tightening, chest pain, shortness of breath, sweating and skin flushing, heart palpitations and tingling, burning or numbness around the lips or in the mouth.

Artificial Colors:

This list is seemingly endless, but just look for any color followed by a number in the ingredients. For example, Red No. 3. The only reason these ingredients are added to food and beverages is to modify the color. They provide absolutely no nutritional value, just visual appeal.

Unfortunately, many of these artificial ingredients can be found even in foods and beverages that are supposed to be good for us. For instance, there are sports/fitness/energy drinks that contain several of these ingredients. Meal replacement bars and shakes also include some of these bad additives. I was even fooled into buying a loaf of whole-grain bread only to find out later that it contained an artificial sweetener and this wasn't even a diet or low-carbohydrate version.

Since I began implementing minor adjustments in my food and beverage intake, my weight and body composition have been very easy to maintain, my energy levels are incredible and constant, my mental/emotional state is clear and vibrant, my workouts are easier and I no longer get nagging hunger pains. Although these are only superficial results, they lead me to firmly believe that a lot of good is also happening inside my body.

I encourage you to make some changes in your own diet and see what happens to your body, mind and spirit. You will be making a positive change that will benefit you and your family. Remember, you are the gatekeeper to your own body. It is your responsibility to screen the foods and drinks that you and your family consume. Just because a product is readily available on store shelves does not mean it is good for you.

CHAPTER SEVEN:
Water, Oil, Fiber and Salt
-- A Trainer's Secret Ingredients

How Your Drinking Water Can Kill You

There was a time when I was desperately searching for a restroom every 20 minutes. This condition was not the result of a problem with my bladder or kidneys. I was just drinking too much water throughout the day, mistakenly believing it was going to get me closer to my fitness goals.

There are people who usually have a bottle of water with them as they go about their daily activities, which is sensible. There are other people who carry one-gallon jugs of water with them wherever they go, representing significant overkill. It doesn't take a science degree to figure out what is logical and what is not. In the real world, it is not possible to be running to a restroom every 20 minutes and not many workplaces would tolerate the need to take such frequent breaks. Requiring this many restroom stops can present problems in any type of daily schedule, not to mention placing undue stress on the kidneys.

As a matter of fact, too much water in a short period of time can kill you. Albeit this is an extremely rare scenario, but it does occur. On the other hand, not drinking enough water can also be harmful. Some sources say the human body can survive without water for two to five days, depending on other environmental factors that are present. Personally, I do not want to test any of these extreme theories about how much or how little water can be dangerous. However, there is valuable insight to be gained from knowing what happens at the extreme ends of the water intake spectrum and it is important to find an ideal place in the middle to gauge our own daily water intake.

The middle range will vary from person to person. We have all seen the "eight glasses a day" recommendation espoused by various sources as the most suitable amount. While this amount may be right for some people, it may not be the best quantity for others. You may feel better drinking 12 to 15 glasses per day, while someone else may do just fine consuming six glasses. There are numerous individual factors to consider, but it's important to remember that drinking only one or two glasses per day is simply not enough. This low level of water intake may cause problems ranging from body aches and pains to constipation.

The earth's surface is about 71 percent water and the human body is comprised of between 70 and 75 percent water. Some would say this is a genuine coincidence, but others would not. I believe there is a bigger reason for this and that it is no small coincidence.

No matter what the subject, there are stacks of research papers and articles from a long list of people who can sway our opinion either in favor or against the popular view. The same is true when it comes to research about water. Ongoing debates focus on how much water we should consume, how often we should drink it and from what sources we should obtain it. In the end, it still comes down to each individual deciding what is best for him or her. This is another classic example of where you should rely on logic, common sense or good old intuition to guide you toward the proper decisions.

Tap water or purified? Carbon-filtered or ozonated? The choices are endless and the marketing, combined with media profiles of the pros and cons of numerous types of water, can leave you confused and unable to decide which is the best choice. There are no right answers to these questions. They just give you another opportunity to demonstrate your logic.

That being said, there are a few things you must know about this life-saving gift from nature that we call water. First and foremost, you should know what's in your tap water. Here's why…

In the early 1990s, a water treatment plant mishap in Milwaukee, Wisconsin allowed Cryptosporidium to contaminate the city's tap water for one week. An estimated 100 people died and over 400,000 experienced fever, abdominal cramping and diarrhea - the telltale signs of cryptosporidiosis. It should be noted that most of those who died already had weakened immune systems before drinking the water.

Cryptosporidium is a parasite that lives in the intestines of humans and animals. When human or animal waste products containing Cryptosporidium find their way into the public water supply, the results can be deadly.

This is only one of many potential water supply contaminants. Here are four more common offenders you should be aware of:

* Disinfection Process Byproducts - These are the harmful compounds created when chlorine combines with decaying grasses, leaves and other organic materials

* Arsenic - I'll bet you thought arsenic was only used in murder mystery stories or talked about in bizarre news reports of people trying to secretly kill someone with this hard-to-detect mineral. The truth is our drinking water contains arsenic,

but most people just don't know about it.

* Turbidity - This simply describes the condition of water when decaying grass, plants, clay and other offensive materials become suspended in the water. Disease-causing organisms can latch onto these materials and side-step the disinfection process. When turbidity levels rise, public utility services are supposed to treat the water to make it safe for consumption. However, sometimes it is hard to detect early enough and can lead to increased cases of gastrointestinal illnesses and conditions.

* Lead - According to the Environmental Protection Agency (EPA), water consumption accounts for about 20 percent of our exposure to the toxic metal known as lead. Accumulated buildup of lead in the human body can damage the kidneys, red blood cells and even the brain.

Although the use of lead in household plumbing systems and public water treatment plants was banned in the 1980s, it still exists in old homes, buildings, underground pipe systems and holding tanks. The EPA claims that lead is still used illegally in some cases.

Now, some of this may sound unrealistic to you, but I assure you it is quite real. The good news is that the chance of you dying from ingestion of your tap water is relatively slim. However, I'm sure you would like to get a report of exactly what is in the water being piped into your home and your body.

Here's how to get that information.

If you get your water from a public water supply, you can call your provider or go to the appropriate Web site. Request the latest Consumer Confidence Report, which will tell you where your water comes from and whether your water supply meets the standards as regulated by the EPA. Also, request a printed summary of the levels of over 80 contaminants that the EPA has set limits on.

If your water is supplied by a well, it is up to you to get it tested. You can get a list of certified testing labs by calling the EPA Safe Drinking Water Hotline at (800) 426-4791.

Bottled Water - A Better Choice or Just a Hoax?

There are several variations of bottled water. Take a look in the water section of your supermarket and you will see the following varieties: purified, drinking, spring, mineral, sparkling and distilled.

Taste and texture aside, there are actual quality differences among the various types and brands of bottled water. Stay tuned and I'll tell you the one thing you need to know in order to be sure you are drinking the good stuff.

First, I want to share an interesting piece of information. A water bottling company can get its water from a city's municipal water system, treat it by filtration or disinfection, bottle it and then wrap it in a label with an outdoor nature scene and market it with very minimal disclosure on the label.

Guess what P.W.S. stands for?

Public Water Supply!

How many people do you think actually catch that?

Now, I'm not saying that bottled tap water is bad. Actually, most of it is good. As consumers, however, we should know exactly where our bottled water comes from without having to hunt for the information.

Here's what you can do to ensure you are getting high-quality bottled water. Go with brands that are members of the International Bottled Water Association (IBWA). Look for the IBWA letters on water bottle labels. The bottling plants of IBWA members must remain open to unannounced, third-party inspections by NSF International, an independent certification agency.

However, it is important to note that if a company does not display the IBWA letters on its bottles, it does not necessarily mean the water is inferior. It just means they have chosen not to join the association. Furthermore, there are companies that are not members of the IBWA that produce water that exceeds IBWA standards.

To learn more about these organizations and your bottled water, go to www.bottledwater.org and www.NSF.org. Also visit www.insidethebottle.org.

What I just shared with you is only the tip of the iceberg. When it comes to the discussion of human water consumption, the more research you do - the more consumed you can get by the details. I'm in favor of staying informed and up to date, but I don't lose sleep over the finer details of water safety and quality.

Here is what I do. If tap water tastes good to me, I drink it. I also enjoy the convenience of bottled water and the clear taste of purified or filtered water. I'll even drink distilled water on occasion. Some would argue that vital nutrients are lost in the purification or distillation process, but if you're drinking water from a variety of sources, including tap water, this should not be a problem. You can even add a pinch of sea salt to your water or other drinks to provide a touch of natural electrolytes during those hot summer workouts.

Ever wonder why it feels good to take a shower or bath and how going for a swim energizes you? This is supposed to happen and it's as natural as why you use water to keep yourself clean. Water carries molecules, ions and minerals that interact with your physiology to elicit positive responses. Now, picture the same thing happening as water flows through your internal systems. The requirements of water by the human body are still not fully understood, but your life certainly depends on this liquid.

One last note. Some experts say you can only count straight water toward your daily water consumption. This never made sense to me because most beverages are made of 98 percent water or something close to that. So, I always include my healthy beverages in my daily water quotas and I've always been perfectly hydrated by doing this.

For example, I consider a few servings of green tea or Atlasjuice™ to be part of my water intake. See www.Atlasjuice.com to download your free e-guide, "The Insider's Guide to Optimal Health and Fitness Hydration."

This is good news for people who do not like the taste of plain water because your daily quota does not have to come solely from water. As I have gotten older, my desire to drink straight water has diminished. Don't get me wrong, I still drink a decent amount of it at certain times.

However, I find myself "not being in the mood" for water,

but still being thirsty for something with a little flavor and substance - without adding 135 unnecessary calories to my daily caloric intake. This is why I created Atlasjuice for me, my family and some of my clients.

I am planning on making Atlasjuice available to all loyal Joey Atlas clients in late 2009. Visit the Atlasjuice web site to get on the early notification list for the official release date.

Improve Your Fitness and Sex Life with Olive Oil

Growing up in an Italian household gave me an early, insider's perspective on the health benefits of olive oil. This smooth substance with the greenish-yellow hue was treated like gold in our kitchen. My grandparents would always buy the maximum allowable amount when their favorite brand was on sale at the local supermarkets. Everyone in my family was encouraged to put olive oil on our food because it was good for us.

Looking back, I realize how right my grandparents and parents were. More than 30 plant compounds found in olive oil are believed to serve as strong antioxidants and anti-inflammatory agents which have been known to prevent cancer and improve heart health. Entire books have been written about the positive benefits of olive oil. Even a simple online search for olive oil will provide enough information to make you want to include it as part of your everyday diet.

Olive oil also gives you that wonderful feeling of being satisfied after you have eaten a good meal and will keep you from overeating if you are keeping an eye on your caloric intake. It is equally helpful for individuals who are trying to gain weight because they can boost their caloric intake by 20 to 35 percent just by putting this oil on their salads, vegetables and smoothies.

As I'm writing this chapter, I'm starting to crave olive oil. Even though I'm working in my office, it's easy for me to open a three-ounce pouch of tuna fish, pour in a tablespoon of olive oil, and lunch is ready.

The ideal type of olive oil is organic, extra virgin. If organic is not available, then just go with extra virgin olive oil. There are many different brands from which to choose, so have fun tasting the slight variations among the oils from various countries.

No, I didn't forget about the sex life part. The more fit you are, the better your sex life can be.

Beverly Whipple, professor emerita at Rutgers University and secretary general of the World Association for Sexual Health, explains the connection between sex drive and the good fats - monounsaturated and polyunsaturated - found in olive oil, salmon and nuts.

"You need fat to produce your hormones," said Whipple, who is also a certified sexuality educator and best-selling author. "Cholesterol is metabolized in the liver and you get your testosterone and estrogen, which you need for your sex drive."

If making olive oil an essential part of your diet makes you stronger and healthier, then it is easy to see how your sex life might improve. As a bonus, remember olive oil is great for massages, too, because it is non-toxic and completely edible. You will have to use your own imagination here…

Fiber for Fat Loss and Health

If dietary fiber is essential to good health, then why are so many people not getting the suggested daily allowance of fiber? The answer is easy. There are so many convenience foods that have little or no fiber content. All of the foods we are supposed to be eating for good health and weight control are the ones that contain fitness-promoting fiber. Naturally, if you are eating the typical fast foods and packaged foods as part of a high-calorie, low-nutrient diet, it's easy to see why you are not getting enough fiber.

The recommended daily amount of fiber is 25 grams for women and 38 grams for men. Now, here is the challenge. For someone who is trying to lose weight, it can be tricky to keep their caloric levels in the zone that promotes weight loss while simultaneously meeting the optimal level of fiber intake.

One of the easiest ways to achieve both goals is to use ground flax seeds, preferably organic, in some of your foods. For example, you can sprinkle a tablespoon over your salad or add it to your cereal. You can even sprinkle flax seeds onto an egg or into a smoothie.

Here are a few good reasons to include ground flax seeds in your daily diet. They are conducive to optimal digestion and contain both soluble and insoluble fiber. They are a great source (though not as good as wild salmon) of Omega-3 (polyunsaturated fatty acid), known for reducing the risk of stroke and heart disease. Finally, they have a high concentration of lignans, powerful phytoestrogens that may offer protection against hormone-sensitive cancers.

In addition to the clinical benefits of flax seeds, they also give you that satisfied feeling after a meal and can keep hunger pains at bay for hours.

Pregnant women and women taking certain drugs should check with their physician before taking any form of flax. It is also wise to talk to a pediatrician before adding flax seeds to your children's foods.

Besides adding your own flax to your foods, there are many products -- from hot and cold cereals to multi-grain breads and cookies -- that already contain flax seeds for added health benefits. One product that we like and give to our kids is Flax Cookies from Voortman of Canada, one of the first companies to go trans fat-free. These cookies are carried by Publix in the Southeastern part of the United States. Information about the company is available at www.voortman.com.

Regardless of whether you eat products that contain flax seeds, you will naturally be giving yourself a higher level of daily fiber if your diet is comprised of the proper foods. Depending on your specific daily caloric needs, though, it may be difficult to get all of your fiber, if you are trying to maintain your weight. There are many other types of fiber supplements, but you want to be sure that you go with natural choices without artificial sweeteners, fillers or binders if you need to add them to your diet.

If you are meeting your daily fiber needs but are still experiencing constipation, a great natural remedy you should talk to your doctor about is Super Dieter's Tea. The active ingredient comes from the senna leaf. While the dieter name is misleading, this caffeine-free tea comes in several flavors and has come in handy for me and some of my clients on several occasions. Information can be found at www.LaciLeBeau.com.

Salt - The Evil Condiment and Its Fitness-Promoting Twin

If you have high blood pressure or a condition related to it, you should consult your physician before making any adjustments to your diet after reading this section.

Let me get right to the point by noting there are two types of salt. The first is table salt, the one you already know about, and the other is sea salt. Table salt is mined on land and then goes through a process of refinement, cleansing and mixing. This process leaves you with plain old sodium chloride, devoid of valuable minerals, such as potassium, calcium or magnesium, that function as crucial electrolytes in the body. To make the picture even more grim, this table salt is treated with chemicals and combined with an anti-caking agent to make it easier to pour. This is the salt that leads to health problems.

Sea salt, on the other hand, comes from the ocean and is minimally processed. It retains natural minerals that function as electrolytes in your body and contains some essential trace minerals, as well. Sodium is essential for human life and it makes sense to obtain it from a natural source that supports many functions of the body.

This coincides with my philosophy about fitness nutrition. Everything we need to function at a level of optimal health exists on earth. The foods that were put on this earth to support life were created with absolute perfection. Let me remind you this was not an accident and it did not happen by chance. Therefore, it is incumbent upon each of us to make sound nutritional choices by selecting foods that are as unrefined and unprocessed as possible. This is why I am a firm believer in the benefits of organic foods and ingredients.

CHAPTER EIGHT:
28 Days to Life -- The Blow-Torch Fat-Loss "Diet"

First, let me emphasize that I use the word "diet" to refer to a way of eating rather than a way of NOT eating. As a general rule, most women who are trying to achieve fat loss and weight maintenance should consume between 1,300 and 1,600 calories per day, while men require between 1,600 and 1,900. This is only a generalization and the number may differ in your particular case, but these numbers are good starting points. Actually, the numbers are based on years of working with clients and reviewing historical evidence from the most successful diet programs.

The success of the "blow-torch" concept is based upon the reality that most people unknowingly overeat and sometimes knowingly without admitting it. It is quite easy to consume more calories than you need in a given 24-hour period and much harder to stay within a reasonable caloric range.

The blow-torch eating plan will put you in a proactive mode without any gimmicks, pay-by-the-month special diet food programs or hard-to-find ingredients. Follow the plan as a general guideline and feel free to alternate the various meals. If you stay within the caloric range I propose in the plan, your body's internal "blow torch" will continuously burn unnecessary fat so it will not accumulate on or in your body. After a few weeks (or sometimes in just days), your stomach will shrink and your hunger pains, if any, will decrease. This is a signal that your body is getting closer to where it wants to be and your energy levels will be more consistent and generally elevated.

When eating, do not eat subconsciously. That is, be aware of the bites you are taking and enjoy each bite. Enjoy every taste of what goes into your mouth. By doing this, you will give your body and mind a chance to give you the "OK, that's enough" signal before you reach the bloated and uncomfortable feeling that occurs after you have eaten too much. Overeating equals weight gain and under-eating or eating just enough equals fat loss and maintenance of ideal body weight.

Always ask yourself, "Is what I'm about to eat or drink in line with my goals and is it going to get me closer to where I want to be in terms of how I look and feel?" Answer this question honestly, act accordingly and you will guarantee your success. This is an example of eating in a conscious mode rather than destructive eating subconsciously. Eventually, you will reprogram your subconscious to operate in a mode that is in line with your true goals, values and desires.

If you have a bad day, don't worry. Tomorrow is another opportunity to resume the program. Just focus on pre-planning your needs for the next day to minimize the possibility of any further setbacks.

At least once a day, look at yourself in the mirror from head to toe and say to yourself, "This is working and I can feel and see the changes slowly occurring. I'm on my way and there is no stopping me." You must realize that taking actions to look as good and feel as healthy as possible is one of the most unselfish acts you can perform. Others may disagree, but here is the truth. If you neglect yourself by overeating, drinking and avoiding consistent exercise, you are putting your health and life at risk.

As you age, you will become frail and dependent upon others for the most simple tasks. This is extremely selfish because your poor habits will cause you to become a burden on your loved ones.

Following the Blow-Torch "Diet" is one of the most sensible actions you can take for yourself and your loved ones. This "way of eating" is designed to be easily followed for the rest of your life, whether you are at home, at work, visiting friends or on vacation. Many, if not all, of the foods are readily available at most supermarkets or on the Internet.

Whenever possible, choose organic foods over non-organic. There is no need for me to rehash my beliefs about the benefits of organic nutrition. However, I will remind you that a diet consisting of 55 percent organic foods is better than a 30 percent organic diet and a 30 percent organic diet is better than a 15 percent one. You get the idea.

For every food I list in the Blow-Torch "Diet" - if it is not organic, there is most likely an organic equivalent. A quick search on the Internet will let you know what organic products are available and where you can purchase them.

If there is a specific meal or snack that you do not like, just substitute one that you like, but pay attention to the calories. If you really like a specific breakfast, lunch or dinner, there is nothing wrong with eating it five or six days in a row.

Review the suggested meals for each day and see what happens when you consistently follow the plan week after week. Once you understand how many calories your body requires and which foods are healthy, you can modify the plan to suit your own tastes. The eating plan includes meals that total between

1,670 and 1,900 daily calories for men. Women should keep their caloric intake between 1,300 and 1,600 by simply cutting the olive oil servings to one tablespoon at each meal or going lighter on the snacks. For everyone following the plan, only eat a mid-morning snack if you are hungry. Don't just eat for the sake of eating. Eat only when you are hungry.

For people interested in muscle/weight gain, this plan can still be followed. However, there should be an emphasis on increasing daily calories instead of restricting them.

For vegetarians, feel free to make appropriate substitutions when necessary. The key is to pay attention to calorie levels, while ensuring a balanced intake of protein, high-quality carbohydrates, essential fats and fiber.

When I refer to canned vegetables, I mean the 16-ounce size. And by all means, if you want to use fresh or frozen organic vegetables, that would be ideal. Likewise, if you think the diet does not include enough meat, make the necessary substitutions to suit your taste, but don't forget to count calories.

Regarding alcohol, it all comes down to calories at the end of the day. If you have a glass of wine or one beer, substitute it for your evening snack. Drink sparkling water in social settings and hold off until later if you are going to order a drink. This creates the likelihood that you will drink less.

Why this "diet" works...

While I don't claim to be a nutritional genius with some breakthrough discovery, I have been smart enough to pay attention to several essential factors:

1 - The types of foods that have been put on this earth for optimum life support;

2 - The psychology of how we relate to food;

3 - The actions that result from the psychology of how we relate to food;

4 - How the body prefers to be fueled;

5 - How certain foods satisfy hunger for hours without over-consumption of calories;

6 - People want simple, easy and fast ways to prepare meals;

7 - The general population does not get educated about proper nutrition and the appropriate mindset;

8 - The more a person's diet gets "cleaned up," the more benefits are experienced in other areas of life. For example, more energy leads to consistent exercise and better moods and this positive chain reaction leads to better fitness, health, self-esteem, productivity, relationships, etc…

In a nutshell, these eight points summarize why the diet works. As you may have noticed, I made no mention of magical power foods, secret combining methods or mysterious foods that melt fat. All of the great foods that have been put on this earth for us have inherent magical powers and the ability to burn health-destroying, unnecessary body fat. It becomes a matter of us making these foods a regular part of our life so that they can work their own magic.

Before I reveal the "diet," I want to give you a list of my favorite bedtime snacks as I will be referring to this list throughout the daily meal plans.

Lots of press has been given to the tactic of stopping one's daily food consumption at a certain evening hour. Some say 6 p.m., some say 7 p.m. and some say 8 p.m. If you research the topic, you will find all sorts of "reasons" for this tactic. While I have nothing against this strategy and admit that it does work for some people, I am not a big proponent of it.

Here's why. In my experience - I have found that most people are "calorically challenged" in the evenings, meaning they have a tendency to want to eat more at the end of the day. Therefore, trying to cut off one's food supply when the night is still young becomes more of a challenging diet technique instead of a natural management of total daily calories, regardless of the time of day or night.

Of course, for people seeking to gain weight to add sexy, healthy curves and muscle tone to an overly skinny or scrawny body, you have nothing to worry about here. However, if you are one of the many who are interested in reducing body fat and body weight, then here is my advice.

Don't worry about stopping your food intake at a specific time in the evening. First, see if you can make progress by focusing on management of total caloric intake in the course of a full day. If you find that you need an extra dose of structured discipline, then go ahead and set a cut-off time for your evening calories, but feel free to drink some health-promoting tea in the evening hours with a pinch of stevia. For some people, this is enough to control the appetite.

OK, time to move on…

For bedtime snacks, I have created what I refer to as "My Secret Seven." Of course, you do not want to eat all of these before you go to bed, but you can combine a couple of them as long as you keep the total calories close to 200.

I give you these first as a warm up of sorts before I reveal the "diet."

Here are the seven somewhat indulgent bedtime snacks:

"My Secret Seven"

1. Two tablespoons of NATURAL peanut butter:
-- 200 calories
-- 16 grams of fat (all healthy fat)
-- 9 grams of carbohydrates
-- 7 grams of protein

2. Low-Moisture, Part-Skim Mozzarella String Cheese Sticks (Two):
-- 160 calories
-- 10 grams of fat
-- 2 grams of carbohydrates
-- 16 grams of protein

3. Cashews (¼ cup):
-- 180 calories
-- 15 grams of fat (healthy fat)
-- 9 grams of carbohydrates
-- 5 grams of protein

4. Dried Figs (¼ cup):
-- 110 calories
-- 0 grams of fat
-- 26 grams of carbohydrates
-- 1 gram of protein
-- 6 grams of fiber

5. Fresh or Frozen Blueberries (1 cup):
-- 90 calories
-- 1 gram of fat

-- 21 grams of carbohydrates
-- 1 gram of protein
-- 6 grams of fiber

6. Soy Nuts, roasted & lightly salted (1 ½ ounces):
-- 195 calories
-- 9 grams of fat (very health fat)
-- 13 grams of carbohydrates
-- 16 grams of protein
-- 4 grams of fiber

7. Dark Chocolate (my favorite), (1 ounce):
-- 170 calories
-- 11 grams of fat
-- 16 grams of carbohydrates
-- 1 gram of protein
-- 2 grams of fiber

The bedtime snacks are scrumptious enough to entice anyone to try the rest of the blow-torch eating plan. And now, let's get started so you can see how easy it is to eat healthy meals and to stay within a desired calorie range.

Before you take the next step I want you to know this: By the 28th day of this "diet," you will experience positive changes in your energy levels, the way your clothes fit, what the scale shows, your level of body fat and so on…

But more importantly, by the 28th day, you will have learned what it means to "eat right" and be in complete control of managing your nutrition so that it is completely in line with your values, goals and intentions.

You will answer your own question of "What do I do after the

28th day?" You will know the answer because you will have experienced it for 28 straight days. In other words, you will just keep doing what you just learned. It's that simple.

Now, one last extremely important note before I pull back the curtain to reveal the "diet." At the request of one of my fitness colleague confidantes, I set out to find a Registered Dietitian who would put the Blow-Torch Diet under a microscope to see if it could stand on its own merits as a well-balanced, sensible and safe eating plan. When I decided to do this, I vowed to go "top shelf" with the level of professional I would choose to execute the task of doing an official analysis of my diet.

Staying true to my word, I found someone affiliated with one of the top health/medical institutions in the world who accepted the assignment. Because of a conflict of interest, I am not at liberty to mention the name of the institution, but I will tell you who she is.

Her name is Jillian McMullen, RD,LD/N and her Web site is www.JillianRD.com

She reviewed my "diet" and submitted her recommendations, both general and specific. In order to avoid tainting the originality of the eating plan, I have included Jillian's exact words as a section you can read at the end of the "diet" section.

And now the "diet:"

Day 1.

Breakfast
• Coffee or tea prepared any way you prefer (no more than 100 calories total)

• 1 serving of Kashi GoLean Crunch cereal. (If you prefer to use another brand, be sure to look for high-fiber, high-protein cereal with no artificial sweeteners, such as Aspartame, Nutrasweet, Equal, Splenda, Sucralose or Acesulfame Potassium.)

• ½ Cup of Skim Milk, preferably organic

Mid-Morning Snack (only if you are hungry)
• 1 ounce of peanuts

• 1 cup of strawberries

• 1 cup of green tea with a pinch of stevia extract and a teaspoon of organic whole cane sugar if you like it sweet (you can have this even if you are not hungry).

Lunch
• 1 can sweet green peas (no salt added), water drained

• 2 tablespoons of olive oil

• Salt & pepper to taste

• 1 medium orange or apple

• 12 ounces of sparkling water (see www.LacroixWater.com for an example).

Mid-Afternoon Snack (only if you are hungry)
• 1 part-skim Mozzarella string cheese stick (portion control is easy because they are individually wrapped)

• 3 or 4 dried plums (or prunes)

• White tangerine tea (check out www.RevolutionTea.com, one of my favorites) with a pinch of stevia extract and a teaspoon of organic whole cane sugar if you like it sweet (you can have this even if you are not hungry).

Dinner
• 1 large egg soft or hard boiled or poached or four ounces of chunk light'tuna in water'or ½ can of garbanzo chick peas OVER:

• 3 cups of chopped romaine lettuce or mixed baby greens

• 2 tablespoons olive oil and 3 tablespoons balsamic or red vinegar

• Salt & pepper to taste

• 12 ounces of water

Pre-Bedtime Snack
Select from "My Secret Seven"

Day 2.

Breakfast
• Coffee or tea prepared any way you prefer

• 1 hard or soft-boiled egg with salt & pepper

• 1 small slice whole-grain bread toasted with a teaspoon of butter (yes, real butter!) or you may substitute any 1 medium-sized fruit for the slice of bread

Mid-Morning Snack

• 1 ounce of almonds

• 1 cup of blueberries or raspberries, frozen or fresh with no added sugar

• 1 cup of green tea with a pinch of stevia extract and a teaspoon of organic whole cane sugar if you like it sweet (you can have this even if you are not hungry).

Lunch

• 1 can green beans (no salt added), water drained

• 2 tablespoons of olive oil

• Salt & pepper to taste

• 1 ounce of cheddar cheese or part-skim Mozzarella cheese

• 1 medium orange or apple

• 12 ounces of water

Mid-Afternoon Snack

• 1 ounce peanuts

• 3 or 4 dried plums or prunes

• Earl Grey tea with a pinch of stevia extract and a teaspoon of organic whole cane sugar if you like it sweet (you can have this even if you are not hungry).

Dinner

• 1 large egg, soft or hard-boiled or poached or four ounces chunk light tuna in water or ½ can garbanzo chick peas OVER:

• 2 cups chopped tomatoes and baby carrots

• 2 tablespoons olive oil and 3 tablespoons balsamic or red vinegar

• Salt & pepper to taste

• 12 ounces of water

Pre-Bedtime Snack
Select from "My Secret Seven"

Day 3.

Breakfast
• Coffee or tea

• Whole rolled oats cooked with water, one serving

• 1 tablespoon raisins

• Cinnamon to taste

• 1 tablespoon natural peanut butter

Mid-Morning Snack
• 1 two-ounce nutrition bar. Look for a bar that has around 200 calories with at least 4 grams of fiber and at least 6-8 grams of protein. Remember, no artificial sweeteners (check out www.ThePureBar.com)

• 1 cup of green tea

Lunch

- ½ can sweet green peas and ½ can sweet yellow corn (no salt added), water drained

- 2 tablespoons olive oil

- Salt & pepper to taste

- 1 medium orange or apple

- 12 ounces of water

Mid-Afternoon Snack

- 1 part-skim Mozzarella string cheese stick

- Small/medium banana

- White tangerine tea or tea of your choice

Dinner

- 4 ounces of salmon or other fish grilled, baked, broiled or pan-seared

- 3 cups chopped Romaine lettuce or mixed baby greens

- 2 tablespoons olive oil and 3 tablespoons balsamic or red vinegar

- Salt & pepper to taste

- 12 ounces of water

Pre-Bedtime Snack

Select from "My Secret Seven"

Day 4.

Breakfast
• Coffee or tea prepared any way you prefer

• 1 or 2 eggs, scrambled in olive oil or poached with salt & pepper to taste

• 1 grapefruit or orange

Mid-Morning Snack
• 1 two-ounce nutrition bar that has approximately 200 calories with at least 4 grams of fiber and at least 6-8 grams of protein. Remember, no artificial sweeteners

• 1 cup of green tea

Lunch
• 1 can mixed vegetables without potatoes (no salt added), water drained, steamed or sautéed

• 2 tablespoons olive oil

• Salt & pepper to taste

• 1 medium pear

• 12 ounces of water

Mid-Afternoon Snack
• 1 cheddar cheese stick

• 1 ounce raisins (one box)

• Black tea (visit www.RevolutionTea.com for choices)

Dinner
• 8 ounces of steamed sugar snap peas (in the pod), sprinkled with one tablespoon parmesan cheese

• 2 cups mixed baby greens

• 2 tablespoons olive oil and 3 tablespoons balsamic or red vinegar

• Salt & pepper to taste

• 12 ounces of water

Pre-Bedtime Snack
Select from "My Secret Seven"

<u>Day 5.</u>

Breakfast
• Coffee or tea

• Multi-grain Cheerios, one serving with a tablespoon of ground flax seed

• ½ cup skim milk

Mid-Morning Snack
• 1 ounce cashews - roasted & salted are OK

• 2 or 3 dried figs

• 1 cup green tea

Lunch
- 3 ½ ounce can chunk light tuna in water

- ½ cup baby carrots

- 2 tablespoons olive oil

- 2 tablespoons balsamic vinegar

- Salt & pepper to taste

- 12 ounces of water

Mid-Afternoon Snack
- 2-ounce chocolate bar (dark or milk). (Yes, you read that correctly. Come on, we have to live a little. Just be sure you don't "double dip" on this one for your pre-bedtime snack.)

- 1 cup green tea

Dinner
- 8 ounces of sautéed mixed vegetables (broccoli, corn, zucchini, etc.), sprinkled with one tablespoon parmesan cheese
- 2 cups mixed baby greens

- 2 tablespoons olive oil and 3 tablespoons balsamic or red vinegar

- Salt & pepper to taste

- 12 ounces of water

Pre-Bedtime Snack

Select from "My Secret Seven," but no chocolate tonight. Try dried plums instead.

Day 6.

Breakfast
• Coffee or tea

• 1 mini whole-grain or multi-grain bagel. (If you can't find mini bagels, have half of a regular size bagel)

• 1 pat of butter (yes, real butter)

• 1 tablespoon natural peanut butter

Mid-Morning Snack
• 1 ounce soy nuts

• Medium orange (a convenient alternative is the pre-packaged mandarin oranges in single servings cups -- no peeling, no mess and they do not have to be refrigerated. I learned this one from my kids.)

• 1 cup green tea

Lunch
• 3 ½-ounce can salmon (the best that we've had is the Kirkland Signature Brand from Costco Wholesale, but there are many others available, as well.)

• ½ cup chopped tomatoes, any variety

• 2 tablespoons olive oil and 2 tablespoons balsamic vinegar

- Salt & pepper to taste
- 12 ounces of water

Mid-Afternoon Snack
- 1 part-skim Mozzarella string cheese stick

- 3 or 4 dried plums (prunes)

- 1 cup green tea

Dinner
- ½ can garbanzo beans (chick peas), lightly crushed with a fork

- 2 cups mixed baby greens or romaine lettuce with a tablespoon of ground flax seed

- 2 tablespoons olive oil and 3 tablespoons balsamic or red vinegar

- Salt & pepper to taste. Also try a little onion powder & garlic powder

- 12 ounces of water

Pre-Bedtime Snack
Select from "My Secret Seven"

Day 7.

Breakfast
- Coffee or tea

- 1- or 2-egg omelet with chopped green onion (the long, skinny one) cooked in:

- 1 tablespoon olive oil and 1 pat of butter

- 2 tablespoons of any salsa of your choice

Mid-Morning Snack
- 1 ounce walnuts or peanuts

- Medium peach or nectarine

- 1 cup green tea

Lunch
- Medium garden salad with romaine and/or spinach

- ½ cup chopped tomatoes

- ½ cup cucumber

- Chopped red onion, optional

- 3 tablespoons any variety of shredded cheese

- 2 tablespoons sunflower seeds

- 2 tablespoons olive oil and 2 tablespoons balsamic vinegar

- Salt & pepper to taste

- 12 ounces of water

Mid-Afternoon Snack
- 1 part-skim Mozzarella string cheese stick

- 1 medium apple or medium pear
- 1 cup green tea

Dinner
- 1 Health Valley (or equivalent brand) instant soup in a cup. (These come in convenient single-serving cups. Look for the bean/vegetable variety for better amounts of protein and fiber. They have a great organic line of products.)

- 1 medium cucumber, chopped with:

- 1 tablespoon olive oil

- 2 tablespoons vinegar

- 1 tablespoon of ground flax seed

- Salt & pepper to taste

- Also try a pinch of some green seasonings, such as parsley, basil, etc.

- 12 ounces of water

Pre-Bedtime Snack
Select from "My Secret Seven"

Day 8.

Breakfast
- Coffee or tea

- Organic Optimum Zen Cereal from Nature's Path, one serving. If you prefer to use another brand, choose one with a

high-fiber, high-protein content with no artificial sweeteners
• Skim milk (preferably organic) ½ cup

Mid-Morning Snack
• 1 ounce roasted or raw sunflower seeds

• ¼ cup raisins

• 1 cup green tea

Lunch
• 1 medium whole-grain wrap

• 2 or 3 slices of roasted turkey, chicken or ham

• 1 tablespoon shredded cheddar

• 2 tablespoons of salsa of your choice

• 1 medium orange or apple

• 12 ounces of water

Mid-Afternoon Snack
• 2 kiwi fruits or one fruit of your choice

• 1 tablespoon of almond butter

Dinner
• 4-ounce can of wild salmon in water or ½ can garbanzo beans over:

• ½ chopped cucumber and one medium tomato with a

tablespoon of ground flax seed

• 2 tablespoons olive oil and 3 tablespoons balsamic or red vinegar

• Salt & pepper to taste

• 12 ounces of water

Pre-Bedtime Snack
Select from "My Secret Seven"

__Day 9.__

Breakfast
• Coffee or tea

• 1 scrambled egg with salt & pepper & one tablespoon salsa

• 1 small slice whole-grain bread toasted with a teaspoon of butter

• Or you may substitute any one medium-size fruit for the bread

Mid-Morning Snack
• 1 ounce cashews

• 1 cup blackberries (frozen or fresh with no sugar added)

• 1 cup green tea

Lunch
• 4-ounce can light tuna in water

• ½ can asparagus (no salt added), water drained with a

tablespoon of ground flax seed
- 2 tablespoons olive oil

- Salt & pepper to taste

- 1 small banana

- 12 ounces of water

Mid-Afternoon Snack
- 1 cup fresh or frozen berries

- 1 rounded tablespoon natural peanut butter

- 12 ounces of water

Dinner
- 6-ounce chicken (dark or white meat) baked, grilled or pan-seared OVER:

- 2 cups chopped tomatoes and baby carrots mixture

- 2 tablespoons olive oil and 3 tablespoons balsamic or red vinegar

- Salt & pepper to taste

- 12 ounces of water

Pre-Bedtime Snack
Select from "My Secret Seven"

Day 10.

Breakfast
- Coffee or tea

- 1 cup multi-grain Cheerios with a tablespoon of ground flax seed

- 1 tablespoon raisins

- Cinnamon to taste

- ¾ cup skim milk

Mid-Morning Snack
- 1 two-ounce nutrition bar

- 1 cup green tea

Lunch
- ½ can sweet green peas and ½ can sweet yellow corn (no salt added), water drained 2 tablespoons olive oil

- Salt & pepper to taste and 1 tablespoon parmesan cheese

- 1 pear

- 12 ounces of water

Mid-Afternoon Snack
- 1 serving of granola/trail mix of your choice

- Blueberry tea from Celestial Seasonings, hot or cold

Dinner

- 4 ounces of flounder or other fish grilled, baked, broiled or pan-seared

- 3 cups chopped romaine lettuce or other lettuce

- 1 chopped green onion

- 2 tablespoons olive oil and 3 tablespoons balsamic or red vinegar

- Salt & pepper to taste

- 12 ounces of water

Pre-Bedtime Snack
Select from "My Secret Seven"

Day 11.

Breakfast
- Coffee or tea

- 1 or 2 eggs poached or boiled, hard or soft with salt & pepper to taste

- 1 grapefruit or orange

Mid-Morning Snack
- 1 two-ounce nutrition bar

- 1 cup green tea

Lunch
- 1 can mixed vegetables without potatoes (no salt added),

water drained, steamed or sautéed
- 1 ounce of cheese of your choice

- 2 tablespoons olive oil

- Salt & pepper to taste

- 1 medium peach or nectarine (or other fruit)

- 12 ounces of water

Mid-Afternoon Snack
- 1 tablespoon peanut butter

- 1 ounce dried cranberries or other dried berry

- Tea of your choice

Dinner
- 8 ounces of steamed sugar snap peas (in the pod) sprinkled with one tablespoon parmesan cheese and 2 tablespoons marinara, tomato & basil or hot & spicy Italian sauce. (Gia Russa brand is awesome.)

- 2 cups mixed baby greens

- 2 tablespoons olive oil and 3 tablespoons balsamic or red vinegar

- Salt & pepper to taste

- 12 ounces of water

Pre-Bedtime Snack

Select from "My Secret Seven"
Day 12.

Breakfast
- Coffee or tea

- 2 slices Ezekiel Bread toasted, one with Olivio (found in the butter section) and

- 1 with your choice of nut butter (peanut, almond, etc.)

Mid-Morning Snack
- Soybeans, preferably organic & non-GMO, roasted & salted is OK

- 2 or 3 dried figs (4 or 5 if they are small)

- 1 cup green tea

Lunch
- 5-ounce tear pouch chunk light tuna (see Starkist varieties) ½ cup baby carrots with a tablespoon of ground flax seed

- 12 ounces of water

Mid-Afternoon Snack
- 10 Hershey's Kisses (it's perfectly fine to splurge once in a while.) Just be sure you don't double up on this one for your pre bed-time snack.

- 1 cup green tea

Dinner
- 1 serving of Freschetta's Brick Oven Pizza - Five Italian

Cheeses, Fire Baked Crust. Find it in the frozen food section of your supermarket. (This is the best frozen pizza I've ever tasted.) - make sure you get the square one.

• 2 cups mixed baby greens

• 1 tablespoon olive oil and 2 tablespoons balsamic or red vinegar

• Salt & pepper to taste

• 12 ounces of water

Pre-Bedtime Snack
Select from "My Secret Seven"

Day 13.

Breakfast
• Coffee or tea

• 1 mini whole-grain or multi-grain bagel

• 1 pat of butter

• 1 tablespoon natural almond butter

Mid-Morning Snack
• 1 ounce walnuts or hazelnuts

• Medium peach or orange

• 1 cup green tea

Lunch

- 3 ½-ounce can salmon, any variety

- ½ cup chopped tomatoes, any variety

- 1 tablespoon olive oil and 2 tablespoons balsamic vinegar

- Salt & pepper to taste

- Add to small or medium whole-grain, high-fiber wrap. Roll and eat

- 12 ounces of water

Mid-Afternoon Snack

- 1 part-skim Mozzarella string cheese stick

- 1 cup fresh or frozen (defrost in microwave or let sit on counter) blueberries

- 1 cup green tea

Dinner

- ½ can garbanzo beans lightly crushed with a fork

- ½ cucumber, chopped with a tablespoon of ground flax seed

- 1 tablespoon of raisins

- 1 tablespoon of olive oil and 2 tablespoons balsamic or red vinegar

- Salt & pepper to taste

- Also try a little onion powder & garlic powder

- 12 ounces of water

Pre-Bedtime Snack
Select from "My Secret Seven"

Day 14.

Breakfast
- Coffee or tea

- 1-egg omelet with chopped green onion cooked in:

- 1 tablespoon olive oil

- On top of one slice Ezekiel bread or whole-grain, high-fiber equivalent

- 1 pat of Olivio or butter

- 2 tablespoons of any salsa of your choice (optional)

Mid-Morning Snack
- 1 ounce almonds

- Medium or large grapefruit

- 1 cup green tea

Lunch
- Health Valley fat-free garden split pea soup with carrots. Comes fully prepared as two servings. Just add boiling water to

convenient disposable cup, let sit for five minutes and eat. Eat both servings for a complete meal with only 220 calories total

- 12 ounces of water

Mid-Afternoon Snack
- 1 part-skim Mozzarella string cheese stick

- 1 medium apple or one medium pear

- 1 cup green tea

Dinner
- 1 serving of Freschetta's Brick Oven Pizza - Five Italian Cheeses, FireBaked Crust. Find it in the frozen food section of your supermarket. (This is the best frozen pizza I've ever tasted. Didn't I say that already?)

- 1 medium cucumber, chopped

- 1 tablespoon olive oil

- 2 tablespoons vinegar, any variety

- Salt & pepper to taste

- 12 ounces of water

Pre-Bedtime Snack
Select from "My Secret Seven"

Day 15.

Breakfast

- ½ cup skim milk or 1 cup of tea
- 1 serving of oatmeal with a tablespoon of ground flax seed

- ¼ cup berries of your choice

Mid-Morning Snack
- 6 ounces plain yogurt

- 1 ounce almonds

- 12 ounces of water

Lunch
- Salad of romaine lettuce topped with 3 or 4 ounces grilled chicken or salmon

- 2 clementines or 1 orange

- 12 ounces of water

Mid-Afternoon Snack
- ½ cup cottage cheese topped with pepper and/or one teaspoon ground flax seeds

- 1 apple

- 12 ounces of water

Dinner
- 1 (3 - 4 ounces) grilled or baked chicken breast
- ½ cup barley soup

- ½ cup steamed broccoli

- Small wedge of cantaloupe, watermelon or other seasonal fruit
- 12 ounces of water

Pre-Bedtime Snack
Select from "My Secret Seven"

Day 16.

Breakfast
- Coffee, tea or skim milk

- 1 boiled egg

- 2 slices of turkey bacon

- 1 kiwi or other fruit

Mid-Morning Snack
- ½ cup cottage cheese

- 2 clementines or 1 orange

- Tea or water

Lunch
- 1 (3-ounce) turkey burger on whole-grain or multi-grain bread, one slice or small roll

- Fresh green salad with olive oil
- ½ cup lima beans

- 12 ounces of water

Mid-Afternoon Snack

- ¾ cup baked soy crackers (Genisoy Smart Hearts is a good choice)

- ½ cup cottage cheese

- 1 cup green tea

Dinner
- 1/3 cup red beans and rice, any brand

- Salad of romaine lettuce

- 1 tablespoon olive oil and 2 tablespoons balsamic or red vinegar

- 1 small slice of angel food cake (Time to indulge again)

- 12 ounces of water

Pre-Bedtime Snack
Select from "My Secret Seven"

Day 17.

Breakfast
- Coffee, tea or skim milk

- ¼ cup oatmeal or other multi-grain hot cereal topped with cinnamon and/or a topping of your choice
- 1-egg omelet seasoned to your liking

- 1 small wedge of cantaloupe or other seasonal fruit

Mid-Morning Snack

- Six ounces plain yogurt or a low-fat flavored brand
- 3 or 4 dried plums

- 1 cup green tea

Lunch
- 2 slices of chicken or turkey breast on whole-grain or multi-grain bread with tomato

- 1 apple

- 12 ounces of water

Mid-Afternoon Snack
- 1 cup fresh or frozen berries

- ½ cup cottage cheese

- 12 ounces of water

Dinner
- 1 piece (4 - 6 ounces) of baked cod or other fish

- ½ cup green peas or green beans (no salt added), water drained

- ½ cup low-fat sorbet

- 12 ounces of water

Pre-Bedtime Snack
Select from "My Secret Seven"

Day 18.

Breakfast
• Coffee, tea or skim milk

• 1 slice of whole-grain or multi-grain bread toasted with 1 pat of butter

• 1 soft or hard-boiled egg

Mid-Morning Snack
• 1 ounce of sunflower seeds

• ¾ cup freeze dried or dehydrated fruit (banana, apple, mango, etc)

• 1 cup green tea

Lunch
• 4 to 6 ounces baked salmon or chicken

• Green salad topped with olive oil

• ¼ cup berries of your choice

• 12 ounces of water

Mid-Afternoon Snack
• 8 almonds
• 6 ounces of yogurt

Dinner
• Chicken stir fry with a variety of peppers, onions and

mushrooms
- 1 serving of fruit salad or fruit cocktail

- ½ cup applesauce

- 12 ounces of water

Pre-Bedtime Snack
Select from "My Secret Seven"

Day 19.

Breakfast
- Coffee or tea

- 1 serving of high-fiber, high-protein cereal

- ½ cup skim milk

- 1 orange or other seasonal fruit

Mid-Morning Snack
- 1 ounce roasted or raw sunflower seeds

- ½ cup cottage cheese

- 1 cup green tea

Lunch
- medium whole-grain wrap with 2 slices of roasted turkey, chicken or ham

- 2 tablespoons of salsa of your choice

- 1 tablespoon shredded cheddar

- 1 slice of watermelon or other seasonal fruit

Mid-Afternoon Snack
- ¼ cup raisins

- Fruit of your choice

Dinner
- 1 large stuffed pepper with brown rice, ground chicken or turkey topped lightly with grated cheese of your choice

- Salad of romaine lettuce and your choice of healthy toppings

- 12 ounces of water

Pre-Bedtime Snack
Select from "My Secret Seven"

Day 20.
Breakfast
- Coffee or tea

- 2 slices of turkey bacon

- 1 scrambled egg seasoned lightly to taste

- 1 small piece of fruit

Mid-Morning Snack
- 6 ounces yogurt, preferably plain

- 1 cup blueberries
- 1 cup green tea

Lunch
- Fresh salad topped with thin slices of turkey breast or chicken breast and olive oil

- ½ cup cottage cheese

- 12 ounces of water

Mid-Afternoon Snack
- 1 serving of soy crackers or trail mix

- 1 banana

- 1 cup of tea

Dinner
- 1 pan-seared 4 - 6 ounce tuna steak

- ½ cup barley or other healthy soup of your choice

- ½ cup steamed cauliflower or similar vegetable with 1 pat of melted butter

- 12 ounces of water

Pre-Bedtime Snack
Select from "My Secret Seven"

Day 21.

Breakfast

- Coffee or tea
- 1 serving of oatmeal topped with a tablespoon of ground flax seeds and ½ banana

- 1 grapefruit

Mid-Morning Snack
- 1 pretzel rod

- 1 apple

- 1 cup green tea

Lunch
- 4-ounce can light tuna in water

- 1 tablespoon olive oil and 2 tablespoons rice wine vinegar

- ½ cup lima beans

- 1 apple

- 12 ounces of water

Mid-Afternoon Snack
- 6 ounces of yogurt

- ½ cup carrots or cucumber with sea salt and pepper

1 cup of green tea

Dinner
- Burger made of ground turkey or chicken

- 3 - 4 ounces ½ cup vegetable soup
- Fresh salad with romaine lettuce and olive oil

- 1 small slice of angel food cake

- 12 ounces of water

Pre-Bedtime Snack
Select from "My Secret Seven"

Day 22.

Breakfast
- Coffee or tea prepared any way you prefer

- 1 serving of Kashi GoLean Crunch cereal. (Try Honey Almond Flax)

- ½ cup of skim milk, preferably organic

Mid-Morning Snack (only if you are hungry)
- 1 ounce of cashews

- 1 cup of grapes or cherries

- 1 cup of green tea with a pinch of stevia extract and a teaspoon of organic whole cane sugar if you like it sweet (you can have this even if you are not hungry).

Lunch
- ½ can butter beans (no salt added), water drained

- 2 tablespoons of olive oil

- Salt & pepper to taste (try some garlic powder and onion powder, too)

- 1 medium orange or apple

- 12 ounces of sparkling water

Mid-Afternoon Snack (only if you are hungry)
- 1 ounce mixed nuts

- 3 or 4 dried plums (or prunes)

- Black tea (check out www.RevolutionTea.com, one of my favorites) with a pinch of stevia extract and a teaspoon of organic whole cane sugar if you like it sweet (you can have this even if you are not hungry).

Dinner
- Kashi - Lime Cilantro Shrimp - in frozen food section - can be cooked in oven 3 cups of chopped romaine lettuce or mixed baby greens

- 1 tablespoon olive oil and 2 tablespoons balsamic or red vinegar

- Salt & pepper to taste
- 1 kiwi fruit

- 12 ounces of water

Pre-Bedtime Snack
Select from "My Secret Seven"

Day 23.

Breakfast
• Coffee or tea prepared any way you prefer

• 1 Thomas' whole-grain mini bagel with1 tablespoon of Smuckers natural peanut butter (it comes in an organic version)

Mid-Morning Snack
• 1 ounce of pecans or walnuts

• 1 cup of blueberries or raspberries, frozen or fresh with no added sugar

• 1 cup of green tea with a pinch of stevia extract and a teaspoon of organic

• whole cane sugar if you like it sweet (you can have this even if you are not hungry).

Lunch
• ½ can cooked lentils

• 2 tablespoons of olive oil

• Salt & pepper to taste

• Garlic powder & onion powder to taste

• 1 medium orange or apple

• 12 ounces of water

Mid-Afternoon Snack
• 1 organic Z bar (chocolate brownie) from Clif – these are for kids, but I eat them all the time (proof that I still haven't grown up)

• 3 or 4 dried plums or prunes

• Tea of your choice – be daring here – the choices are endless with a pinch of stevia extract and a teaspoon of organic whole cane sugar if you like it sweet (you can have this even if you are not hungry).

Dinner
• 8 – 12 sautéed shrimp

• Baked zucchini and/or yellow squash with sea salt, pepper, garlic powder and onion powder

• 1 cup chopped tomatoes and baby carrots

• 2 tablespoons olive oil and 3 tablespoons balsamic or red vinegar

• Salt & pepper to taste

• 12 ounces of water

Pre-Bedtime Snack
Select from "My Secret Seven"

Day 24.

Breakfast
• Coffee or tea

- 1 serving raisin bran cereal with a tablespoon of ground flax seeds

- Cinnamon to taste

- 4 - 8 ounces of skim milk

Mid-Morning Snack
- 1 two-ounce nutrition bar. Look for a bar that has around 200 calories with at least 4 grams of fiber and at least 6 - 8 grams of protein. Remember, no artificial sweeteners (check out www.ThePureBar.com)

- 1 cup of green tea

Lunch
- 1 can organic lentil soup from Health Valley (no salt added) Sea salt & pepper to taste

- 1 medium orange or apple

- 12 ounces of water

Mid-Afternoon Snack
- 1 cheddar string cheese stick (or similar)

- Small/medium pear or apple

- White/green tea or tea of your choice

Dinner
- 4 ounces of grouper or other fish grilled, baked, broiled or pan-seared

- 3 cups chopped red leaf and/or green leaf lettuce

- 2 tablespoons olive oil and 3 tablespoons vinegar of your choice

- Salt & pepper to taste

- 12 ounces of water

Pre-Bedtime Snack
Select from "My Secret Seven"

Day 25.

Breakfast
- Coffee or tea prepared any way you prefer

- 1 or 2 eggs, scrambled in olive oil or poached with salt & pepper to taste

- 3 tablespoons salsa of your choice

Mid-Morning Snack
- 1 two-ounce nutrition bar that has approximately 200 calories with at least 4 grams of fiber and at least 6 - 8 grams of protein. Remember, no artificial sweeteners
- 1 cup of green tea

Lunch
- 1 serving (flat can) sardines in water

- 2 tablespoons olive oil

- Salt & pepper to taste

- 1 medium pear or apple

- 12 ounces of water

Mid-Afternoon Snack
- 1 rounded tablespoon almond or cashew butter

- 1 ounce raisins (one box)

- Black tea

Dinner
- 1 serving organic white cheddar macaroni and cheese

- 2 cups mixed baby greens or lettuce and 1 chopped tomato

- 1 tablespoon olive oil and 3 tablespoons balsamic or red vinegar

- Salt & pepper to taste

- 12 ounces of water

Pre-Bedtime Snack
Select from "My Secret Seven"

Day 26.

Breakfast
- Coffee or tea

- One serving multi-grain cereal of your choice, hot or cold with a tablespoon of ground flax seed

• 4 - 8 ounces skim milk

Mid-Morning Snack
• 1 ounce cashews or sunflower seeds - roasted & salted are OK

• 1 cup melon of your choice or other fruit

• 1 cup green tea

Lunch
• 3 ½-ounce can chunk light tuna in water mixed with

• 1 chopped cucumber

• 2 tablespoons olive oil

• 2 tablespoons balsamic vinegar

• Sea salt & pepper to taste

• 12 ounces of water

Mid-Afternoon Snack
• 2-ounce chocolate bar (dark or milk). (Yes, again!)

• 1 cup green tea

Dinner
• 8 ounces of sautéed baby corn, water chestnuts and chopped carrots, sprinkled with one tablespoon Romano cheese

• 2 cups mixed baby greens with one tablespoon of sunflower seeds

- 2 tablespoons olive oil and 3 tablespoons balsamic or red vinegar

- Salt & pepper to taste

- 12 ounces of water

Pre-Bedtime Snack
Select from "My Secret Seven," but no chocolate tonight. Try dried plums instead.

__Day 27.__

Breakfast
- Coffee or tea

- 1 whole-grain waffle with half a banana

- 1 pat of butter (yes, real butter)

- 1 tablespoon natural peanut butter

Mid-Morning Snack
- 1 ounce soy nuts or roasted peanuts

- Medium orange (a convenient alternative is the pre-packaged mandarin oranges in single servings cups -- no peeling, no mess and they don't have to be refrigerated. I learned this one from my kids.)

- 1 cup green tea

Lunch
- 3 ½-ounce can salmon or tuna

- ½ cup chopped tomatoes, any variety

- 2 tablespoons olive oil and 2 tablespoons balsamic vinegar

- Salt & pepper to taste

- 1 small or medium apple

- 12 ounces of water

Mid-Afternoon Snack
- 1 granola bar - see Back to Nature Chewy Trail Mix Bars at www.BackToNatureFoods.com

- 1 orange or other fruit

- 1 cup green tea

Dinner
- ½ can black beans with one tablespoon shredded cheddar cheese on top of

- 2 cups mixed baby greens or romaine lettuce

- 2 tablespoons olive oil and 3 tablespoons vinegar of your choice
- Salt & pepper to taste. Also try a little onion powder & garlic powder

- 12 ounces of water

Pre-Bedtime Snack
Select from "My Secret Seven"

Day 28.

Breakfast
• Coffee or tea

• Hot whole-grain cereal of your choice - see Quaker's organic line, Kashi's Go Lean Hearty All Natural and Organic Blueberry Almond from Target. These cook within minutes on your stovetop and can be made the day before to take to work the next day. No excuses!

• Add a half cup of berries of your choice

Mid-Morning Snack
• 1 ounce pistachios

• Medium peach, nectarine or apple

• 1 cup green tea

Lunch
• ½ avocado chopped and tossed with

• ½ cup chopped tomatoes

• ½ cup cucumber
• Chopped red onion, optional

• 3 tablespoons any variety of shredded cheese

• 2 tablespoons sunflower seeds

• 2 tablespoons olive oil and 2 tablespoons balsamic vinegar

- Add Mrs. Dash seasoning of your choice - original, garlic herb, extra spicy, etc.

- 12 ounces of water

Mid-Afternoon Snack
- 1 nutrition bar - about 200 calories

- 1 medium apple or medium pear

- 1 cup green tea

Dinner
- 1 serving Tabatchnick Tuscany Lentil Soup (see www.tabatchnick.com) sprinkled with 2 tablespoons of grated cheese of your choice

- 1 medium cucumber, chopped with:

- 1 tablespoon olive oil

- 2 tablespoons vinegar

- 1 tablespoon of ground flax seed

- Salt & pepper to taste
- Also try a pinch of some green seasonings, such as parsley, basil, etc.

- 12 ounces of water

Pre-Bedtime Snack
Select from "My Secret Seven"

The best personal trainers and fitness consultants teach their clients and students how to become their own trainers. By giving you this 28-day sample "way of eating," my primary objective is to show you what four weeks of wise nutrition looks like with the ultimate goal of you taking the information and making changes, if necessary, to suit your specific needs. Along the way, you will naturally learn what foods and meals work with your lifestyle and schedule. It is quite possible that the 28-day program will be exactly what you are looking for and the meals will suit your needs and preferences. If so, great. Take it and run with it.

I have taken liberties to mention certain brands in many of the meals. Take this as information being passed between two friends in everyday conversation and not as product endorsements. These just happen to be products that we enjoy and at the same time, fit into the Blow-Torch way of eating.

Let me remind you that while I suggest you derive most of your nutrition from organic sources, I am aware of the obstacles you may face regarding availability and price. To this, I say do what you can and just know that with every passing month the availability and price factors of organic foods and beverages will continue to become less prohibitive.

With more organic/natural-themed stores opening, such as Whole Foods and Trader Joe's, and with traditional supermarkets, such as Publix and Shop-Rite, devoting more shelf space to organic items, access to lower-priced organics will soon be a reality.

While the plan outlined on the preceding pages may not be suited for vegetarian diets or gluten-free diets, it can easily be modified to suit both needs. Individuals following a vegetarian or gluten-free diet should know how to remove the foods that do not fit their needs and substitute the ones that do. The key is to do this while staying within the recommended caloric ranges and maintaining a balanced intake of complex carbohydrates, proteins and fats.

Hence, my answer to the longstanding question: "What am I doing wrong? I follow an extremely healthy diet, but I cannot lose a pound."

There is a massive difference between eating healthy and eating healthy while not taking in more calories than your body needs. Even too many healthy calories will lead to weight gain or prevent weight loss. Healthy eating also means eating the right amount of food. Doing so will ensure you have enough energy to exercise and explore the rock-solid strategies described in the next chapter.

But first - just like I promised, here are Jillian McMullen's professional recommendations for the Blow-Torch "Diet:"

General Suggestions

* Breakfast coffee or tea, prepared any way you prefer- I caution you to put this amount of freedom on a sample menu. Many people may interpret this the wrong way and feel that it is OK to go to Starbucks and order a high- calorie/high-fat venti-sized (that's 24 ounces) coffee. How about specifying that they keep it below 50-100 calories from sweeteners and added cream? (for example, a pinch of stevia with a teaspoon of organic whole cane sugar and 1 tablespoon of skim milk or 2 tablespoons of fat-free creamer).

* I feel that 2 tablespoons of olive oil is too much at any meal.

I teach my clients that 1 teaspoon of oil is a serving of fat. On some of the days, there is as much as 4 tablespoons of olive oil in one day (480 calories and 56 grams of fat just from olive oil!) I know that this additional fat can help stave off hunger, but I think it would be more balanced to decrease the servings to 1 tablespoon of olive oil and add 1-2 ounces of lean protein instead. Lean protein can also help to ward off hunger.

For example: **Lunch for Day 1:** decrease olive oil to 1 tablespoon and add 1-2 ounce pre-cooked roast chicken breast (or other meat) to the peas.

* **Snacks:** Nut butters like peanut butter and almond butter are great for snacks. However, I would always pair it with something that they can realistically spread it on. (I personally love eating peanut butter right out of the jar, but I don't know many other people that are willing to do it!). Below I've included examples for specific snacks where this is the case.

* You do a great job at including the appropriate caveats and reminding readers that they can mix-and-match the meals if they prefer a specific breakfast, etc. I also like that you caution those on salt-restricted diets to speak with their physician first. However, I would also put in a caveat for diabetics…especially when it comes to eating chocolate since this can be a lot of sugar at one time for them.

* Since you speak a lot about "choosing the right caloric amount for you," this may be a good time to suggest the client seek a registered dietitian to determine their caloric needs or visit a credible Web site such as www.mypyramid.gov to determine their needs. In my experience, many people think they need an outrageously low amount of calories in order to lose weight, only to end up feeling hungry all of the time and

then get quickly discouraged. I used to work with an Indirect Calorimeter, which was a great tool to show people that "yes, your body burns more than 500 calories a day!" On the flip side, there are also those who think they need *way* more calories than what they actually need and may aim for the higher end of your range only to maintain or even gain weight.

* Overall, I really enjoyed reading your book. The menus show the reader that it is possible to eat healthy without spending a ton of time in the kitchen preparing and cooking meals. Depending on how comprehensive you want to get with it, you may want to include some type of guideline or reference for restaurants. Many restaurants have their menus with nutrition facts online. But again, it just depends on how much you want to get into it. I would definitely refer my clients to this book. It answers many questions I get asked all of the time.

<u>Specific Suggestions From McMullen:</u>

* Day 1 and 19 Breakfasts: Add specific guidelines for choosing a cereal if they do not want to use Kashi GoLean (choose a cereal without artificial sweeteners, greater than 3 grams of fiber per serving, less than 8-10 grams of sugar per serving)

* Day 8 Mid-Afternoon Snack: Instead of 2 kiwis with 1 tablespoon of almond butter try:
    -1 small apple or 1 small banana with 1 tablespoon of almond butter OR
    -2 kiwis with 1 ounce almonds

* Day 9 Mid-Afternoon Snack: Instead of 1 cup fresh or frozen berries and 1 rounded tablespoon of natural peanut butter try:
    -1 cup fresh or frozen berries topped with 1 ounce slivered

almonds and 1 tablespoon fat-free whipped cream
OR
    -1 small apple or 1 small banana with 1 rounded tablespoon natural peanut butter

* Day 11 Mid-Afternoon Snack: Instead of 1 tablespoon of peanut butter and 1 ounce of dried cranberries try:
    -1 ounce peanuts and 1 ounce dried cranberries

* Day 12: While splurging should definitely be taught to our clients, "moderation" also needs to continually be emphasized. Ten Hershey's Kisses might lead to unwanted afternoon "crashes" since this is a lot of sugar and no nutritional value. How about 5 Hershey's Kisses (preferably "special dark") and a piece of fruit? Oranges or 1 cup of strawberries would pair nicely with chocolate....

* Day 16, 18, and 20 Lunches; Day 21 Dinner; and Day 25 Breakfast: Fresh Green Salad with olive oil, scrambled eggs in olive oil...I would continue to specify quantities (i.e. fresh green salad with 1 tablespoon olive oil).

* Day 25 Lunch: Cut 2 tablespoons of olive oil down to 1 tablespoon of olive oil and add 5 Triscuits (or whole grain cracker) for the sardines.

* Day 25 Mid-Afternoon Snack: Instead of 1 rounded tablespoon of almond or cashew butter and 1 box of raisins try:
    -1 box raisins OR 1 ounce cashews or almonds
    -1 rounded tablespoon cashew or almond butter and 4 dried apricots (nut butters are tasty spread on dried apricots!)

* *I love Day 25 Dinner!!*

* Lunch Day 28: I would definitely cut back on the olive oil since they are also getting healthy fat from the avocado.

Jillian McMullen, RD, LD/N
Nutrition Consultant
www.jillianrd.com

CHAPTER NINE:
Seven Rock-Solid Principles
To Deliver You to Fitness

By this stage in the game, you should be starting to develop a renewed mindset about how you can accomplish your fitness objectives by taking the proper steps. You should firmly believe that you can transform your body and your overall health by exercising on a regular basis and making smart food choices. It is now time to turn up the heat and proceed with seven definitive principles designed to move you from where you are today to where you want to be tomorrow.

No. 1: Express Gratitude, Admit Acceptance & Proclaim Desire --

Gratitude is easy to achieve because it simply means being thankful for the gift of life you have been given, regardless of your current circumstances and level of fitness.

Acceptance acknowledges where you are at this particular moment in your life, but it must also include the realization that you possess the power to change your state of mind and your subsequent level of fitness.

When I refer to desire, I mean deciding whether or not you want to live your life to the fullest. This is your opportunity to take charge and proclaim your desire to achieve as many goals as possible in your life.

No. 2: Be Realistic in Your Goals --

You have said your thanks, you are at peace with where you

are and you have expressed your desire to make the most of yourself and to get the most out of life by living as fit and healthy as you reasonably can. Setting realistic goals will help you channel your desire into actions that have intent and direction. Create your goals not as specific numbers or dates, but more as ranges or zones. For example, vowing to lose 11 to 16 pounds in the next two to three months is much more realistic than trying to lose 14 pounds in five weeks. The same type of logic can be used for people trying to gain weight.

It is fine to use outside examples as fuel for motivation, but your true progress must be measured relative to yourself. Let's use the "celebrity body" as an example. You can think of many celebrities or athletes, both male and female, who would be considered to be in great physical condition. Even in these high-profile groups, however, we will find many different versions of a fit body. The point is not to get your heart fixed on a genetic structure that you cannot achieve, but rather to move yourself into the optimal zone of your own genetic range by being, feeling and looking the best you possibly can. In other words, unleash your own potential rather than trying to mirror someone else's physique.

Keep in mind that your goals should be more than just superficial ideals. In addition to weight, clothing sizes, body fat and what you see when you look in the mirror, you also want to address things that are found in a typical medical checkup, such as blood pressure, cholesterol and triglyceride levels to name just a few.

No. 3: Find the Things You Like and Consistently Stick with Them --

There are endless options and choices when it comes to exercise programming. Your main focus is to find a few things that you like to do and then continue doing them on a regular basis. Once you are comfortable with your current exercise program, feel free to add some variety by injecting new material into your regular routine. One of the keys to your success is consistency, better described as assimilating your fitness and nutrition regimen into your daily life so they become a natural part of how you live.

It is easy to be distracted by all of the products and programs that are marketed to the public through every possible media outlet. While some of the products and exercises may be legitimate and worthwhile, you cannot do all of them or change what you are doing every other week. This is not safe nor is it conducive to long-term success.

By sticking with what you like the best, it will be easier to keep your program going on a regular basis. For the extreme beginner, this may be joining a basic group conditioning class or just following a beginner fitness video in the privacy of your own home. As your fitness improves and your progress becomes more evident, you may start to look for some variety and more advanced levels of exercise. The key is not to make drastic changes. Be gradual in your transitions and your progress will continue.

For instance, do not stop one activity cold turkey and immediately switch to something else. Keep your first method going and add the new material once or twice per week, being sure to start at a level that is appropriate for you whether you are at the beginner, intermediate or advanced stage.

No. 4: Let Logic and Common Sense be Your Guide --

The allure of so many products on the shelves of every store makes it very tempting for people to take a chance on something that seems like a miracle solution. As a result, the vitamin and diet supplement industry is huge with a capital "H." The problem with the industry is that there are a lot of gray areas, which result in products that are fraudulently marketed, misleadingly labeled and sometimes just downright harmful.

From the small independent shops to the massive international bulk retailers, an endless supply of miracle fixes are marketed to the unsuspecting general public by preying on people's weaknesses and tapping into their emotional pain. The markups are big and the use of radio, television and the Internet to continually market ineffective products to the public is proof that companies are profiting without delivering the advertised benefits.

Fortunately, not all of the supplement industry borders on being fraudulent. There are many upstanding companies with products that are what they claim to be and do what they promise to do. Even so, I do not advocate the unnecessary consumption of various supplements.

The beauty and cosmetics industry also has questionable practices and products. From miracle firming creams and anti-fat/cellulite lotions to body wraps and vibration treatments, the marketing and packaging can be disgustingly humorous when you truly know how the body works.

And, of course, we can't forget the spectrum of absurd fitness gadgets that promise the most ridiculous results. There are far too many to list, but the reality is that nobody will ever burn off body fat simply by wearing a rubber corset or hooking up electrodes to their problem areas.

Whether it is a breakthrough fat-burning herb or some new incredible device, look at what you see through the filters of logic and common sense.

No. 5: Leverage the Power of Wise Nutrition --

For many years, I believed true fitness resulted from doing high-intensity workouts and consuming unnecessary supplements. However, with time comes wisdom if you keep an open mind. I have always kept myself open to learn that the true magic of fitness success happens with wise nutrition. Yes, proper exercise is essential, but to get the results that most people seek, you must use the foods that nature provides in amounts that are conducive to your goals. Nature provides a wide array of healthy foods in the form of fruits, vegetables, nuts, grains, beans and seeds. Doesn't it make sense to eat these natural foods rather than opting for processed items. The earth produces everything we need and from nature should come your first choice of nutrients for optimal life support.

The more our foods are manipulated and processed, the more healthy qualities they lose and the less valuable they are to the human body. Granted, some foods are simply not edible in their raw state, but I'm not referring to those.

I'm a big believer in eating as clean and natural as possible, but doing so can be a bit challenging in today's fast-paced society. As a family, we do the best we can. If there are no fresh, organic vegetables in the house, for example, we always have canned or frozen varieties on hand.

The point I'm trying to make is that you must learn not only about the quantity of calories, but also their quality. You want your foods to be as nutrient-dense as possible with minimal or no elements that may be present as a result of non-organic farming and/or processing and preserving methods.

What you put in your body has a tremendous impact on every aspect of your existence, ranging from how you look and feel to the results of your annual physical exam. The nutrition choices you make throughout each day are a prime factor in both your short-term and long-term fitness. Change doesn't happen overnight, but with gradual modifications you can change your diet so that it works for and with you, instead of against you.

No. 6: Know that Fitness is a State of Being --

Your fitness success is not defined by one workout or one meal, but rather by your overall state of mind. You are human and certain life situations can make you feel less in control and interrupt your regular routine. Maybe you will miss a few exercise sessions because of your work schedule or family issues. You may find yourself in situations where your food choices are less than optimal. The reality is, though, that a few missed workouts and a few bad meals will not obliterate a true fitness lifestyle and mindset.

The "throw in the towel" and "fall off the program" attitudes contribute to the Fitness Failure Epidemic. Many people become angry with themselves for not sticking to a rigid exercise routine or for eating a few meals that are not conducive to fitness and eventually they give in to their emotions. They believe they have failed and begin to question their long-term ability to stick with a healthy program. This cycle seems to drive the annual New Year's Eve resolution frenzy.

The ideal approach to fitness should sound like "This is how I'm going to start thinking," and not "Let me try this program for three weeks and see if it works." Fitness success is not defined by reaching one's ultimate goals, whatever they may be, but rather by where the person stands right now as opposed to where they have been in the past. Let me illustrate.

Ponder the following scenarios and answer the question "Who is experiencing fitness success?"

A sedentary mother of two, who has never exercised, is about 65 pounds overweight, low on energy and lacking self-esteem. She realizes the best thing she can do for her family is to start taking care of herself. To this end, she starts exercising 30 to 40 minutes per day and paying attention to her choices of foods and beverages, making healthier choices and taking note of the quantity and quality of the calories. Each day, she is making progress and feeling healthier, stronger and sexier, even though she has many pounds to shed before her health is in balance.

A male fitness/muscle fanatic spends over two hours in the gym six days per week in addition to working his 9-to-5 weekday job. He spends hundreds of dollars each month on muscle powder formulas and over-hyped supplements. By most people's standards, he appears to be in great shape. In his own mind, he is fearful of what might happen if he cuts back on his workouts and does not eat 35 grams of protein every two hours. In short, his fitness rules his mind and his life, instead of making it better and enhancing it.

Which person is achieving true fitness success? Your answer should clearly point to the mother.

Aim for balance because that is what life should be about. Do not wait; start today. Start working on your thought processes and your state of mind by thinking proactively and not leaving your fate up to your very impressionable subconscious.

Take control of your subconscious by being more conscious of your thoughts and your actions. Draw up your plans, gather your resources, combine the two and get moving. Create your personal version of fitness success and your entire life will benefit. Remember, fitness is not an end result. It is a state of continual being.

No. 7: Be Your Own Personal Trainer --

One of the most repeated statements I've heard from my clients over the years is "I wish you could follow me around all day every day, telling me what to eat and what not to eat."

In essence, they are expressing a desire for a full-time personal trainer under the guise that they do not have the necessary willpower, something that we all possess in unlimited amounts. The difference between people who use their willpower and the people who do not is that the people who use it create enough "want power" to move them into intentional thoughts and deliberate actions.

Professional trainers do this very well. They know how they want to look and feel. They want good health and a high quality of life. They know how they want to be perceived. "Want power" is the precursor to willpower. If you want something bad enough, you call upon your will to make it happen.

Acting as your own trainer, you must define your wants and let them dictate all of your actions. You can press the snooze button on the alarm clock and sleep in or wake up an hour early and complete a good workout program. What do you want more -- an hour of sleep or better fitness? You can eat a high-fat, low-nutrient, calorie-loaded meal or you can eat the type of food that is conducive to your goals. What do you want more -- an energy-zapping meal that provides immediate gratification or a body-benefiting, health-promoting, energy-boosting meal? It's your choice. Be your own trainer and remind yourself about your goals and what you value for yourself and those around you.

Another trait of good trainers is the foresight to pre-plan. Look at the next few days in your schedule. What will you be doing? Are you traveling? Are you entertaining? Do you have a special function to attend? If you are mindful of your schedule, you can plan what you must do in order to stick to your program. If you're going to be traveling, pack your workout clothes and sneakers. If you are going to a party, ask if you can bring the veggie platter and fruit salad. These are just a few examples of the many ways you can implement a proactive mindset similar to that of a personal trainer, who is looking out for your best interests regarding your health and fitness.

Good trainers are also persistent and continual learners. They constantly seek to learn about the body and how it is affected by various elements, food and exercise. They are open to new ideas, if the ideas are logical. They are also creative and make it fun, easy and natural to live a fitness lifestyle.

It wasn't until I became my own personal trainer that I realized how much easier it is to stay committed to a balanced and healthy lifestyle. Becoming my own trainer was an essential stepping stone in helping me get the "fat kid" out of my system once and for all.

Wherever you are starting from, no matter how far you feel you have to go and regardless of what stage of fitness you are at, becoming your own personal trainer will give you the ability to look at yourself from an outside perspective. If you have a good relationship with "your trainer," you will take the advice and make it count every time your trainer advises or reminds you.

In the next chapter, you will learn about your Fitness Success Kit. I put this package of bonuses and support materials together with the intent of giving you the tools you will need in order to become your own personal trainer. Some of the tools will help you with "doing" the right things. Other tools will help you enhance the "thinking" part of your fitness journey. Together, these tools create a powerful combination of the exact devices that will allow you to be your own trainer.

CHAPTER TEN:
The Most Effective Exercise Program for You

I remember meeting a new client for his initial consultation back in the mid-1990s. I asked him the same question I ask all of my new clients. Have you ever exercised before? He replied, "I've been exercising on and off for the last 23 years. I've been off for the last 22 of them."

Besides being a very funny way of telling the truth, his answer underscores the stark reality of so many failed attempts at fitness success. It highlights the fact that most people do not stick with a program for life. There are so many reasons why this problem occurs, but many of them are the result of unrealistic exercise programs that cannot be followed for a long period. Without proper guidance about how to modify a program to fit one's lifestyle, most people give up completely and deny themselves a better quality of life.

From this notion springs the simple fact that the most effective exercise program for you is one that realistically fits into your schedule and lifestyle, so that it naturally becomes an essential part of your life. When I hatched the idea to write this book and get it into your hands, I feared this particular chapter the most, certainly not because I lack the ability to create the right program for your needs, but because of my disdain for presenting an exercise program simply by using static photos.

There is nothing like watching your trainer demonstrate the exact form of each exercise with variations for different users to ensure that you know precisely how to maintain proper form throughout the entire move. This pertains to joint angles, body positioning, range of motion, speed of movement and overall tempo of the entire routine.

The only logical solution and the one that I believe will deliver the most value and high probability of your long-term success was to create an exercise program and deliver it to you via DVD. I was warned not to do this because the DVDs are often stolen in stores, libraries and other venues where people can physically handle the books. It was a valid point to consider, but it did not provide me with a satisfactory answer and so I kept brainstorming.

How would I be able to give you this essential, three-level home fitness DVD?

The most simple and realistic solution I could reach was to create a private web page that you and other clients who invested in this book could visit, sign up for the free bonus DVD, Basic Home Fitness, and have it mailed directly to you for just the cost of shipping and handling. Your private web page is www.YourFitnessBook.com/MyBonusKit. Please do not share this web address with others because anyone who wishes to obtain the DVD without purchasing the book can do so only by paying the full price of $28 plus shipping and handling at www.HomeFitnessDVD.com.

Also included in your bonus Fitness Success Kit:

- Self Assessment Form ($17 value)
- The Cardio Truth Report ($15 value)
- Fitness Success Blueprint ($23 value)
- "Be Fit!" Reminder Poster ($10 value)
- Travel Fitness Cheat Sheets ($11 value)
- Blow-Torch Food-Shopping List ($9 value)
- Web Site Quick Reference Sheet ($9 value)

- Home Fitness DVD Progression Plans ($19 value)
- "Before and After" Coaching Questionnaire ($22 value)
- Inspirational "Before and After" Interviews and Photos ($24 value)
- Secrets of Stretching - The Priceless Rewards of Flexibility ($20 value)
- 2-Weeks Free Members-Only Pass to BestFitnessAdvice.com ($55 value)

That equals $262 worth of life-enhancing fitness tools as my way of saying thanks and delivering on my promise of helping you achieve permanent fitness success. Take advantage of each tool as you journey along your way to a better quality of life.

The essence of this program revolves around the fact that it can be done at home, at the office or on the road. There is no need to travel to a health club or gym, no need to fight the crowds or guess about what you are supposed to be doing. This is not a program for bodybuilders, power lifters or fitness competitors. Created for beginners and individuals who have suffered chronic fitness failures, this program is designed for real people with real families and careers.

It is specifically suited for people who are more interested in a balanced, enjoyable approach to fitness, people who would rather exercise where they want and when they want. This program is not for men looking to gain as much bulky muscle as possible nor is it for women who want to lose every extra ounce of body fat at the expense of their health and overall wellbeing.

Your ideal program is one that you will look forward to because it feels good, not one that you dread because of how hard you must work or because you are extremely sore for several days after each workout. This exercise program is your foundation for long-term sex appeal, total body strength, self-confidence, optimal energy levels, health enhancement, functional flexibility and reduction of aches and pains.

This is the point where I stop writing and direct you to the previously mentioned Web page so you can claim your bonus Fitness Success Kit. Remember, we encourage and welcome "before" and "after" success stories and photos. We look forward to hearing about your success on your journey from fatness to fitness.

As a matter of fact, we will be expecting your complete fitness success story for possible inclusion in my next book, "Fitness - The Atlas Way." An important part of my next book will be a compilation of "before" and "after" success stories from people just like you.

So, take your "before" photos as soon as possible (not just one - take a handful of them), record your measurements and fill out your self-assessment form, as well as the "Before and After" Coaching Questionnaire today. Then, start putting this book and all of the support materials to use and don't look back.

When you believe you have achieved success, send me your complete story (you can use my "Before and After" Coaching Questionnaire as a guideline) and your "before" and "after" photos.

Email them to: success@yourfitnessbook.com

As I mentioned throughout this book, fitness is a state of being - not just something you do occasionally. It's 24/7 and 365 days a year.

It always helps to have little reminders of what your goals and values are to help you stay on the right path. Keep this book where you can see it, where you can easily refer to it and pick it up for support, direction, motivation and inspiration.

I sincerely thank you for letting me into your life and becoming a part of it - just as by reading this book and taking action - you have become an important part of mine.

I'll be waiting to hear from you.

"Don't Be Like Everybody Else…Be Fit!"

-- Joey Atlas

About the Author

Fat Kid Turned Fitness Pro

Challenged by a tendency to gain fat easily and an early obsession with food, Joey's desire to become fit, lean and strong led him to an education and career in fitness. Even as a fitness pro, however, he constantly struggled with the "fat kid" inside.

Joey saw his weight yo-yo between extremes over the course of 15 years until he ballooned up to 168 pounds during one of the most challenging times of his life. That is too much weight for someone who is 5 feet, 2 inches tall.

When his "baggy drawstring sweatpants" didn't fit anymore, he knew it was time to take control. From that day on, Joey realized the secret to permanent fitness success lies within the mind more than anything else.

Busy in the Fitness Business

As he grew personally, Joey was able to use his experience to help hundreds of others who came to him for personal training, nutritional guidance and lifestyle management for improvements in fitness and overall well-being. His clients who embraced the concept of mindset adjustment reaped the long-term benefits of a new way of living.

The success with his clients led to a schedule of 14-hour days working with people on a one-on-one basis. However, he quickly realized this rigorous work schedule was not conducive to his family life and this method of helping others was actually limiting the number of people he could reach. As a result, Joey created a line of fitness DVDs with the intent of helping people all over the world through his simple methods and effective programs.

His first program, *"The Leg, Butt, Hip and Thigh Makeover,"* rolled out with so much success that it wasn't long before his clients were asking for "more, more, more!" He then created six more DVD sets and has several more planned for release this year. Many loyal clients were also asking for a Joey Atlas fitness book. You are holding that book, Joey's first of many to come, in your hands right now.

Food and Values for Fitness Success

A firm believer in clean nutrition, Joey is a big advocate of organic foods and credits much of his own long-term fitness success to giving his diet a thorough, yet simple, makeover.

One of his main mantras is that fitness success is basically guaranteed when the fuel for motivation comes from one's own values - values that are built on the desire to get the most out of the gift of life by living a fitness lifestyle.

According to Joey, logic and common sense are two of the most important elements to maintain in your lifelong journey of fitness success. He reminds you that, "Fitness is not a thing that you do, but rather a state of being."

Web Sites to Facilitate Your Fitness Journey

- Visit www.BestFitnessAdvice.com for your free "52 Fitness Success Tips," and to learn more about Joey's Members-Only Interactive Fitness Magazine Web Site.

- Sign up for your free subscription ($87 value) to Joey's

weekly fitness e-newsletter, ``Secrets of a Trainer'' at www.JoeyAtlas.com.

- Visit these sites for more free exercise instructions and to learn about Joey's Home, Office and Travel Fitness DVD sets:

  www.LegButtHipThighExercises.com
  www.CoreAbdominalExercises.com
  www.BodyWeightLegExercises.com
  www.UpperBodyExercise.com
  www.OptimumFlexibility.com

To inquire about bringing Joey into your organization as a consultant, speaker, mentor or motivator, please send an email to Pam@JoeyAtlas.com with details regarding your project needs or call (866) Yes-Joey or (904) 436-6052.